Balance Exercises for Seniors

Step by Step Fully Illustrated Home Workouts for Fall Prevention, Improved Stability, and Posture

Robert Balazs

LANDSHIP

We're a gang or crew of four manning
this landship, gliding over and trawling
each drill. Inside, the broad-belt rungs
potatoes past to the drop of a hold.

Our hands don't touch the healthy:
only debris, the frost-bitten ones
and last year's progenitors, the globes
of mucus that held until now.

Since lunch, enough pinks to feed a life.
Now our measure is full holds and trailers,
drawing toward farmyard lights. We work
on under a fluorescent lamp, divining.

Standing two aside in our canvas cabin,
lulled as time grows, we are quick
and our eyes have sharpened. Still drawn
by horsepower, nothing stops us

except nature; the hoarfrost or waterlogged ground.
I jump off for a piss as we veer near a hedgerow.
Crows have fled the black bronchiole
and vacated the clots of their own making.

I watch it pass, an ugly sailing junk
lit like a lantern. Voices from inside
warm the din as the tractor tows
the harvester down a dark slope,

to fresh drills. I have found my pitch
in this season of evictions.
A place on a moving belt above earth
with a part scraping it.

Acknowledgements to the Editors of the following publications where some of these poems have appeared: *Kansai Raw* (Japan), *Poetry Ireland Review*, *Cúirt Journal, Japanophile* (USA), *Cyphers, The Irish Times, Windows Publications Monthly, Social Alternatives* (Australia), *The Café Review* (USA), *Connect, Stand Magazine* (UK), *The Gettysburg Review* (USA). *Sailing to Hokkaido, Windows Publications, Poesia tra Sicilia e Irlanda* (Italy) *La Contraddizizione* (Italy) *At the Year's Turning, An Anthology of Responses to Leopardi* (Dedalus Press) edited by Marco Sonzogni.

Thanks to the Tyrone Guthrie Centre at Annamakerrig and the Heinrich Böll house in Achill for stays there.

Worple Press is an independent publishing house that specialises in poetry, art and alternative titles. **Worple Press** can be contacted at 12 Havelock Road, Tonbridge, Kent, TN9 1JE. Tel. 01732 367 466, Fax 01732 352 057, email: theworpleco@aol.com

Titles Include:

The Falls – Clive Wilmer   £6.00   ISBN 0 9530947 3 1
'Clive Wilmer's first book since his *Selected Poems* of 1995 is as seamlessly constructed as the poems themselves. Wilmer's style is cool, formal, crisp and energetic.' *TLS*.
'boldly lyrical, broad in reference, felicitous in the craft of verse...' *Elizabeth Jennings*

Choosing an England – Peter Carpenter   £5.95   ISBN 0 9530947 0 7
'Honest, considered and moving... Peter Carpenter has tied some new marriage knot around post-modernist and mainstream verse... accomplished and hugely enjoyable.'
David Morley

A Ruskin Alphabet – Kevin Jackson   £4.50   ISBN 0 9530947 2 3
'If you have not yet had enough Ruskin, you may like to consult A Ruskin Alphabet, a collection of facts about and opinions on Ruskin and Ruskinites, together with a variety of pithy remarks from the man himself...   **Jim Campbell,** *TLS*

Looking in All Directions – Peter Kane Dufault   £10   ISBN 0 9530947 5 8
'The best poems are engrossing, representative of the best of the American "Wilderness School", with nothing of the Ouija board about them but a real spiritual hunger... there is a wry, detached note that sounds even in his intensely inward-looking pieces. He observes the physical world keenly, and idiosyncratically, and frequently serves the "didactic muse", but he can sing from the heart too.... It is surprising that other publishers have ignored Dufault; but Worple Press have done him proud'.
John Greening, *TLS*

Table of Contents

A Free Gift to All My Readers!

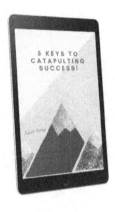 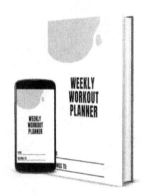

As a thank you and to help you on your fitness journey, I would love to send you a free copy of my weekly planner so that you can plan your workouts, as well as my eBook titled *5 Keys to Catapulting Success!*

To receive your complimentary copies now, please visit *www.robertbalazs.com.*

Exercise Video Companionship

All of the exercises featured in this book are also available to view in video format. Not only is this book fully illustrated, but to give you the best start on your journey to better balance, I have also included a free video companion!

To get your video playlist, please visit *www.tinyurl.com/Rob-Balazs*.

Introduction

If you love life, don't waste time, for time is what life is made up of. –
Bruce Lee

As we approach retirement, we start to look at things that we can enjoy spending our newfound freedom on. Maybe you want to travel the world or finally learn to dance. Perhaps you have always wanted to spend more quality time with your friends, children, or grandchildren. Whatever it is that you are looking forward to, you need your health on your side to be able to accomplish it.

Do you ever feel unsteady on your feet?

Have you felt like the room is moving while you are standing still?

Or have you felt lightheaded or faint?

When we have poor balance, it can be intimidating to take on social engagements, and we end up missing out on some of life's golden moments because we are too scared of the potential of sustaining injuries from falling, especially if we have already felt the effects of a developing balance disorder. Previous bad experiences can dent our confidence and we may feel like we don't want to be a burden on our families, so it would be best if we don't go to celebrations with them. The fear that feeling unstable on your feet will embarrass you or worse, cause an injury, can create a negative cycle where you do less and become more prone to accidents through lack of practice, and then more frightened.

It's important to realize, though, that you aren't alone. These kinds of problems affect many people but can also be resolved with a targeted balance training routine. One in six older Americans has a vision impairment, one in four has loss of feeling in the feet, and three in four have abnormal postural balance testing results (Dillon et al., 2010). This leads to an increased chance of falling, hip fractures, and increasing rates of heart disease and other morbidities. Additionally, balance dysfunctions are reported to physicians by 8 million adults in the U.S. (AGS Health in Aging Foundation, 2022).

The ability to balance requires the healthy functioning of several bodily systems working in coordination with each other seamlessly. It is an ability that we need to consciously learn as toddlers but that soon becomes as natural as breathing as we enter our childhood and adulthood. However, as we continue our journey into our fifties and beyond, balance starts to become something that we need to consciously put effort into again. It can stop us enjoying outings and hobbies, but it can also severely affect our daily routines, making things like shopping for groceries, moving around our homes and even showering a daunting task for some of us.

Poor balance can be the result of many things, from a central dysfunction in the body's balance centers to a lack of strength in the spine's supporting muscles. Poor core stability and recovering from injuries are also common causes. For those of us with pre-diagnosed conditions, we learn to recognize when the signs and symptoms rear their heads, but many people may not even know that a balance problem may be what is causing them to feel unwell or destabilized. The National Institute on Aging suggests that you should look out for the following common signs that could be an indication of a balance disorder:

- staggering while walking

- dizziness

- vertigo

- a feeling that you will fall

- lightheadedness

- a floating sensation

- blurred vision

- confusion

- disorientation

Anyone experiencing a sudden onset of these symptoms should consider speaking with their primary care physician for further investigation. But for many seniors, these kinds of symptoms gradually come on over time or worsen with time so slowly that you may even miss their onset all together or may not have considered associating them with one another.

As an older adult, regular physical activity is one of the most important things you can do for your health. –Centers for Disease Control and Prevention

As we age, it is inevitable that we will become somewhat less active and be less able to maintain healthy systems in our bodies. In America, only 50% of 50–64-year-old's report that they regularly exercise, with just 32% of those 65 or older taking part (Carroll, 2005). It's understandable to be wary about getting more active if you have experienced falls in the past, injuries such as rolled ankles, or have a pre-existing diagnosis of balance dysfunction. However, balance training can help to reinstate your confidence, improve your independence, and, in some cases, even reduce episodes of dizziness. Aging doesn't have to condemn you to a sedentary lifestyle or the inevitability of reduced mobility and accidents. Regular exercise for seniors can help to prevent this decline and even reverse it to a certain extent.

A healthy balance system gives you more energy and strength, and helps you move freely and confidently. –Rob Fox, YMCA fitness teacher

Research suggests that a regular commitment to balance training can bring you the following benefits:

- improved mobility

- improved posture

- increased muscle tone

- increased reaction times

- improved cognitive function

- improved core stability

- improved ability to perceive your body in relation to your surroundings

- reduced instances of falling and injuries

- increased confidence

- increased independence

- increased energy

By following along with the exercises in this book and dedicating just ten minutes a day, you can regain control of your mobility and independence, and feel fitter in the process.

I want to give you the confidence to start experiencing the joys that your hobbies, family, and friends bring you again. In this book, I show you fully illustrated exercises that will develop your key muscles for body stability and train your brain to overcome a dysfunctional ability to compensate for changes in your environment. I also cover how you adapt these exercises to suit your own health and personal goals, as well as how to make the most of equipment specially designed for improving balance.

As always, before the commencement of any sort of exercise routine or regime, please be in contact with your local healthcare provider. This is especially relevant for those with prior injuries or health issues.

Thanks for purchasing my book. After you are finished reading the book, I would really appreciate it if you could help spread the word and leave a review on Amazon so we can reach a greater audience and help them in the same way that we have hopefully helped you. To leave a review, scan the QR code below with your mobile phone and click on the book. Once you have clicked on the book, you will be able to find the button to leave a review. If you do not own a smartphone, please search for my book on Amazon and take 60 seconds to leave a review. You are amazing!

About the Author

Robert Balazs was born in Canada but relocated to Scandinavia by the time he was 19. He has always had a passion for exercise, sports, and helping people.

Today, Robert is a certified personal trainer and has over a decade of experience under his belt. Over this time, he has helped hundreds of clients realize their potential and become pain-free. Helping people to achieve their health goals matters deeply to Robert, who feels it is greatly rewarding to have the privilege of witnessing people's struggles become better over time.

Robert decided to write this book when he realized that, so few seniors actually have any kind of structured exercise or training program in their daily routines. He couldn't understand how so many people were missing out on the numerous benefits of staying active and healthy into and past their 50s.

Wanting to reach and help more people is Robert's main goal in writing this book. He wants the knowledge that he has gained to help other people take control and improve their daily lives.

Chapter 1:

Balance and Its Importance

To understand what may be contributing to your balance concerns, it is important to understand what we mean when we talk about balance and why it is important for us in daily life. The word 'balance' itself refers to our ability to keep ourselves upright when sitting or standing, and our ability to properly sense the position of our bodies in relation to the ground.

When our balance is healthy, we can move around and conduct our daily tasks with little to no conscious thought. When this ability deteriorates, we consider ourselves to have poor balance. Poor balance can manifest in several ways. The symptom that most people fear is the inability to remain on their feet, which results in trips and falls. In the U.S., 3 million older people are treated for fall related injuries every year, and over 800,000 are hospitalized because of those injuries (Centers for Disease Control and Prevention, 2021).

However, trips and falls are not the only signs or symptoms of a balance issue. Other symptoms you may have started to notice include:

- unexplained dizziness

- a feeling as though you are spinning when standing still

- a feeling of floating

- feeling sick (nausea)

- a feeling as though you may pass out

- an inability to stand or sit still without assistance

These symptoms can be very frightening and may last for only an instant or up to a few days at a time. Early symptoms of balance disorders can be signs of other health conditions too. If you experience any of these symptoms for the first time without explanation or if they last more than a few days, you should contact your primary care physician for a check-up.

How Does Aging Contribute to Bad Balance?

Our bodies use several functions at once to maintain a healthy ability to balance. Due to this complexity, there are several dysfunctions that can ultimately cause or worsen balance problems. Good balance requires the normal functioning and coordination of the following bodily systems:

- **Musculoskeletal**: The physical structure of your body, the skeleton, muscles, ligaments, and tendons.

- **Nervous system**: The nerves, spinal cord, and brain.

- Proprioception: The brain's ability to understand the position of your body in space relative to your surroundings.

- **Inner ear balance center**: A collection of small organs within the ear that act as a biological spirit level for the body.

- **Vision**: The eyes, optic nerve, and vision center of the brain.

When we age, our body's natural ability to maintain itself becomes less efficient. As a result, these systems can deteriorate. Problems in each individual system can increase with age, as well as the prevalence of reported balance concerns for seniors.

Worldwide statistics show that nearly 4% of women and 3.5% of men have moderate to severe vision impairment. Those figures rise to nearly 12% and 10.5% of women and men 50 years of age or older (Elflein, 2021).

Nearly 8 million adults in the U.S. report balance problems to their physician, ⅓ of adults over 65 experience falls linked to these problems, and over half of those who are over 75 (AGS Health in Aging Foundation, 2022).

Problems with our muscles and joints can lead to poor posture and an altered stride. This is the most common cause of trips and falls. For seniors, falls are particularly concerning due to the prevalence of such an incident resulting in a fractured hip. More than 300,000 older people are hospitalized each year due to hip fractures (Centers for Disease Control and Prevention, 2021).

What are the Benefits of Exercise to Combat This?

Staying active is a key component to improving balance and preventing falls. Our sedentary lifestyles go against the natural evolution of our bodies and can lead to weakened muscles, poor posture, and loss of coordination.

Studies show that six weeks or more of balance training exercises can reduce the occurrence of lower limb injuries, such as ankle or knee sprains, as well as speed up the healing process after receiving a sprain (McKeon et al., 2008). However, it is recommended to train your balance for at least 11–12 weeks to get the maximum benefit from your exercise. These kinds of studies remind us of the importance of an effective ability to balance and show how the lower limbs in particular can be a crucial part of improving your balance. Muscles that stabilize your ankles and knees, along with core stability muscles in your abdomen and back, must function in perfect coordination to maintain your position when standing or walking. When any of these are working out of sync with the others, the instance of falls increases.

Exercising to improve your balance has several health benefits, including:

- Helping to reduce the effects of aging on balance.

- Improving coordination to better recover from slips and prevent falls.

- Improved posture and reduced posture related pain.

- Improves your walking technique to better handle uneven surfaces, such as walking on gravel or uphill.

- Increasing the strength of muscles.

- Reducing the likelihood of lower limb injuries.

- Improving confidence in standing or walking.

Other Things That Can Help Prevent Falls

Though balance training exercises are important in helping you to become more confident and prevent falling, there are other ways you can improve your safety alongside your exercise program. As we discussed, balance requires the coordination of many functions in your body to work efficiently. We can counter the effects of dysfunction in these areas with proper medical attention from your primary care physician or ophthalmologist. For example, having your eyesight and hearing regularly tested and properly using any glasses or hearing aids provided will help you to have the best possible understanding of your environment while you are moving around it.

Sometimes our balance is affected by drugs. If you are at risk of falling, you should limit the amount of alcohol that you drink, as it can negatively affect your coordination. Besides recreational activities, prescription medication can sometimes have side effects that include dizziness or confusion. It is important that you read all the documentation given to you with your medication to be aware of any such side effects. If a medication is making you feel overly dizzy or sleepy, you should consult your physician to see if they can provide a counter measure, or alternative.

If you require the help of a walking aid, don't be embarrassed to use it, but do be sure that you are aware of the correct way in which it should be used. If you do require the help of a walking aid, you aren't alone, and you certainly aren't any less of a person because of it. 25% of older Americans use either a cane, walker, wheelchair, or scooter (Huffman, 2015).

Health conditions such as diabetes, heart disease, and high or low blood pressure can contribute to falls, so it is important to understand your condition and how it affects you in daily life if you have any additional health needs. It is important to be sure that you stand slowly to prevent a fall in your blood pressure and dizziness. Be sure to get enough sleep too, as feeling sleepy can also contribute to poor balance.

Now that we have covered your health and body, I want to give you some tips on making sure that your environment is as safe as possible and making sure you are properly equipped to handle outside environments too. Keeping your home's walkways clear of clutter is a simple but effective way to make it easier to get around your home safely. If you have any pets, be sure to keep a lookout for them when you are walking through your home and let them go ahead of you where possible to reduce the risk of them causing you to trip.

Your choice of footwear is important both in the home and when you are out and about doing errands. Be sure to avoid walking around the house in socks alone; a good pair of shoes is best. If you absolutely can't live without a cozy pair of slippers, get yourself a pair with a rubber non-slip sole and a style that covers your whole foot. Avoid backless slippers. When choosing your shoes, look for styles that are low-heeled, non-skid, and have a sole that is thick enough to protect you from objects that may be on the floor, but thin enough so that you can still feel the surface beneath your feet. Avoid wearing platform shoes. They may look safe as they don't hold your feet in a high-heel position, but the large sole will stop you from being able to properly sense the position of your feet in relation to the floor.

Whenever you go somewhere new that you are not familiar with, take your time to make your way around. Be extra vigilant when it is icy out or the floor is wet. Both conditions can make the ground very slippery and dangerous. Save some sand and salt so that you can spread it near your front and back doors, or along any paths in your garden to improve the way your shoes will grip the surface.

Chapter 2:

Testing Your Balance

What to Expect From This Book

Who is This Book For?

I wrote this book with the intention of spreading knowledge of how to improve balance and reduce the risk of falling for seniors or anyone who is experiencing a reduced ability to balance following an injury or illness. This book is for all those who want to get ahead with their balance skills, prevent falls from occurring, and increase confidence in their mobility. It can also be a great source of information for anyone who has a loved one with any of the conditions listed above who they want to be able to help.

What Types of Exercises are in This Book?

This book contains exercises aimed at strengthening your muscles and training your balance centers to improve your posture and, in turn, increase your stability while sitting or standing. The exercises are grouped into the following three types:

- Sitting: A great place to start if you fear losing your balance while standing, so that you can still feel safe while developing your posture.

- Standing: Practicing movements that combine to create your walking style and improve your strength.

- Vestibular: Carefully chosen to retrain your balance centers, improving your brain's ability to comprehend how your body relates to the world around you.

All the exercises I have included in this book can be scaled up to really push your ability to the next level, once you have familiarized yourself with the base routines. Similarly, if you have already experienced falls, sustained injuries, or suffered illnesses such as a stroke, which is currently limiting your ability to perform these exercises, can be scaled down so that you can still start to retrain your balance safely.

How to Use This Book?

Before you start any new exercise routine or training plan, you should always consult your primary care physician or other health professional to ensure that it is safe and correct for your individual health situation.

The exercises in this book are intended to be done daily. Choose ten of the exercises each day and keep rotating through them, both to ensure that you target every area of improvement in your balance and to keep things interesting. If you enjoy your routine, you will be more likely to stick to it. Once you feel like you are confident with each exercise, move onto the advanced exercises and consider adding in balance tools to take your training up a notch.

When Should You Train Your Balance?

The key to seeing good results is consistency. Building a routine that you can stick to every day will help you get the most out of your balance training. It is important that you check your diary or planner to select a time of day that you can stick to regularly. Please visit my webpage now to get your free copy of my weekly planner to help you start planning your new routine today (*www.robertbalazs.com*).

Practicing your exercise routine first thing in the morning after you wake up can help to boost your mood and prepare you for the day ahead. Alternatively, planning your routine before bedtime can relieve any tension that you may have built up during the day, helping you relax and get a better night's sleep. Ultimately, you will know which times feel right for you. Don't be afraid to change your time if you feel it isn't right. It is better to change your routine so that you are comfortable and will stick with it, than to feel uncomfortable while you train and ultimately feel like giving up.

Testing Your Balance

Below are four exercises that you can use to test your current ability to balance. They can be used as a tool to measure the improvement in your balance as you progress on your exercise journey. For safety reasons, it is important that you conduct these exercises with a sturdy chair nearby, so that you can grab onto it if you feel yourself starting to lose your balance or feel lightheaded.

How to use these exercises to measure your improvement:

1. Perform each exercise, holding the position for as long as you can before you are forced to correct your posture by moving a foot or arm out to save your balance.

2. Use a stopwatch or other timer to time the length of your hold.

3. Record the times that you get for each exercise.

4. Repeat the exercises once a week and compare your times to the previous week, so that you can see your improvement.

Feet Together Eyes Closed

1. Stand straight with your feet together.

2. Keep your arms by your sides and close your eyes.

3. Hold this position for as long as possible and record the length of time that you can stay here without needing to step aside to rebalance or grab onto a chair or counter.

You will feel your body swaying when your eyes are closed. This is normal, but if you feel yourself starting to fall or feel dizzy, then open your eyes and stop. You may want to take a seat until you feel better.

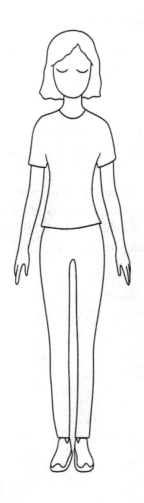

Single Leg Hold

1. Stand straight with your feet together.

2. Keep your arms by your sides.

3. Bend one leg 90 degrees at the knee.

4. Hold this position for as long as possible and record the length of time you can stay here without needing to put your foot back on the floor.

5. For an accurate representation of your balance repeat this with your other leg and record that time too.

Be sure to keep your arms by your sides, avoid the temptation to hold your raised leg with your hand. However, if you feel any pain in your knees or ankles, you should stop this test until you have worked on strengthening your legs.

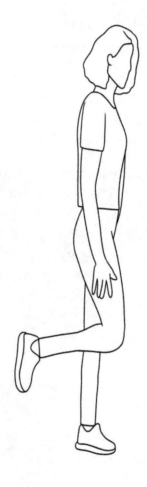

Tandem Stance

1. Stand straight with your feet together.

2. Keep your arms by your sides.

3. Place your right foot in front of your left, bringing your foot to the center line and touching the heel of the right foot to the toes of the left foot.

4. Hold this position for as long as possible and record the length of time you can stay here without needing to step out and regain your balance.

5. For an accurate representation of your balance, repeat this with your left foot in front of your right foot and record that time too.

Be sure to keep your feet on the center line in front of one another, avoiding letting your toes point outwards or stepping too far forward.

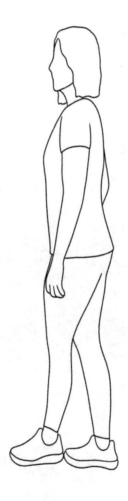

Chapter 3:

Getting Started

Preparing for Success

Equipment Needed

Athletic clothing: Choose clothing that is breathable but not too loose. Cotton or specialist athletic clothes with breathable materials are a good choice. You will want to choose items that allow you to move freely while exercising, but avoid clothing that is too long in the arms or legs.

Appropriate footwear: Either exercise in bare feet or choose a pair of shoes with a flat sole that will support the arch of your foot and ankles. Your footwear should be properly laced or otherwise fastened to prevent it slipping off.

Water bottle: Sufficient hydration is critical to a safe and effective workout. Be sure to keep a water bottle nearby and take regular sips between exercises. You will lose water through your sweat, so drinking enough to replace this will be important.

Chair: You will need to have a sturdy chair handy when exercising. Be sure to choose a chair that is free from any damage and that connects soundly to the floor through all four legs. Look for a chair with a solid seat. A dining chair is a good example. Avoid using a sofa, as this can lead to slouching and a reduced ability to perform the full movement of the exercise.

Towel: Different people will experience different amounts of sweating while they exercise. However much you sweat, it is a good idea to keep a towel handy so that you can wipe it away and stay comfortable.

Music: If you prefer to exercise with music playing, choose some that will keep you motivated or relaxed, to your taste. Whichever music you choose, be sure to prepare it before you start. Getting distracted by choosing or skipping songs mid-exercise can lower your motivation to continue.

What Should Your Exercise Schedule Look Like?

I always recommend that you start out slowly and increase your exercise as you progress along your fitness journey. Balance training can be taxing, so it's best to ease into your full routine in stages. Start with two to three sessions per week. You can add in another session each week until you reach a full daily routine. Remember that exercise should be enjoyable, if you feel pain ease back and take a rest, check that you are correctly doing your technique so that you don't overexert yourself. There is no shame in sticking to just a few sessions a week for as long as you feel you need to, especially if you are already diagnosed with a balance disability (dysfunction) or have an injury.

Where and How to Set Up

The exercises in this book can be performed anywhere, but there are some things you need to consider before getting started. Choose a space to exercise in that has a comfortable temperature and sufficient heating or air conditioning depending on the season. If you feel uncomfortable exercising in front of people, opt for an exercise space that has some privacy.

I recommend avoiding hard flooring such as concrete or tile, but if you can't avoid this, it is fine to counteract this by using an exercise mat or blanket. If you need to use blankets, be sure not to choose thick or layered blankets such as duvets, as they can shift underfoot and negatively affect your balance.

Be sure to clear your exercise space of any clutter before you start. You may also want to ensure that any pets are placed in another room to avoid potential accidents from them getting underfoot.

Before you start, take a moment to get into the correct frame of mind. Build some anticipation for the things you will soon be able to do independently again. Go into your new routine with a winning mindset, and don't forget your water bottle.

The Importance of Breathing

A common mistake that people make while exercising is holding their breath through the movements. This reduces the efficiency of your exercise in several ways. Firstly, it makes you feel out of breath more quickly, but it also limits the amount of movement available for you to use during your exercise around your chest and back. Holding your breath can tighten your muscles and result in poor function as it lowers the amount of oxygen available for them to utilize in movement.

For the exercises I have chosen for you, I recommend consistent and controlled breathing. Keep a regular pace, breathing in through your nose and out through your mouth. If you ever notice yourself holding your breath, stop and take a deep breath in, let it out in a sigh, do this three times, and then restart your exercise. This is intended to refocus you on your breathing. If this is unsuccessful and you find you return to holding your breath, it could be a sign that you are finding exercise too strenuous, and you should consider adapting it to make it easier for yourself until you are able to increase the intensity again.

Warming Up

Warming up before you exercise is a keyway to improve the results of your exercise and reduce the likelihood of injury by preparing your body for the work it is about to do. It gets your blood pumping by increasing your heart rate and starts to transport more oxygen to your muscles so that they are ready to perform for you. It's also a good way of getting you into the right mindset for your exercise routine by triggering the thought that it's time to work out now.

I have included three warm-ups for you that are ideal to prepare your body for balance training. However, if you find them too difficult, they can be substituted for general warm-up techniques such as walking, running, or spinning. If you choose to substitute for any of these more conventional techniques, I recommend that you do them for at least five minutes to sufficiently raise your heart rate and body temperature.

For the warm-ups below, perform each one for 40 seconds—take a 20-second break, and then repeat. Take another break and then move onto the next warm-up. If you choose to incorporate the full routine, it will take you six minutes to complete.

Seated Hip Circles

Areas Targeted: Hips, abdomen, and back muscles; visual input, and proprioception—particularly the balance structures in the ear.

1. Sit in your chair with your feet hip width apart.

2. Place your hands on your hips with your elbows bent out to your sides.

3. Lean to your left and then forwards, rotating your torso above your hips.

4. Move your torso across to the right and back up to a tall, seated position.

5. Repeat the circle for 20 seconds, then switch directions.

6. Lean to your right and then forwards, rotating your torso above your hips.

7. Move your torso across to the left and back up to a tall, seated position.

8. Repeat the circle for 20 seconds.

9. Take a 20-second break and then repeat.

The goal is to draw a circle in the air with your shoulders so that it creates a circular motion around your hips. Try to make your circles as deep as possible but keep your bottom fully on the seat. Avoid curling or arching your back as far as possible. You want to aim to generate the movement from your hips and not your spine. If you feel unsteady during this exercise, you can place your hands on the sides of the chair for support but be sure not to drive the circles from your shoulders if you do this.

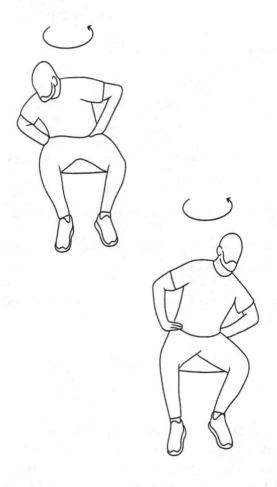

Seated Hip Leans

Areas Targeted: Hips, abdomen, neck, and back muscles, visual input and proprioception—particularly the balance structures in the ear.

1. Sit in a chair with your feet hip width apart.

2. Place your hands on your hips with your elbows bent out to your sides.

3. Lean forwards bending at the hip as far as you comfortably can.

4. Slowly sit up straight.

5. Repeat leaning forwards and back for 40 seconds.

6. Take a 20-second break and then repeat.

The aim of this warm-up is to bend at the hip, avoiding curling your back as you move. To keep the movement controlled throughout, you may want to pause briefly at your furthest point forward and when you sit back upright, this will help you to avoid getting into a swinging motion that is relying on momentum rather than poise. If you find this too difficult, you can support yourself by placing your hands on either side of the chair. If you choose to do this, avoid pushing yourself forward with your arms.

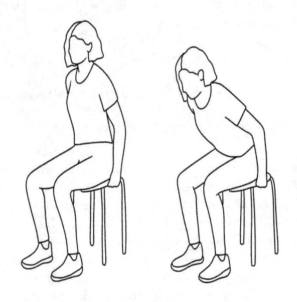

Seated Marches

Areas Targeted: Hips, abdomen, thigh muscles, and proprioception.

1. Sit in a chair with your feet hip width apart.

2. Place your arms down by your sides.

3. Lift your left leg, keeping your knee bent.

4. Lower your left leg, then lift your right leg, keeping your knee bent.

5. Lower your right leg.

6. Repeat this action, alternating from one leg to the other for 40 seconds.

7. Take a 20-second break and then repeat.

Lift your knees as high as you comfortably can but be sure not to allow your legs to fall out to the sides as you do. You will want to alternate as quickly as you can without overexerting yourself, as this exercise is particularly good for raising your heart rate. As with the other warm-ups, if you find this too difficult, you can support yourself by holding either side of the chair. Be sure not to hold your arms rigidly if you do this, as it may encourage you to hold your breath, which you need to avoid doing.

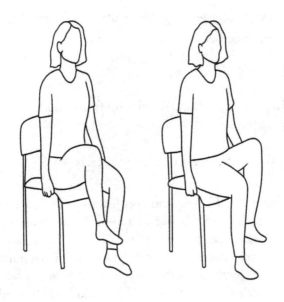

Chapter 4:

Seated Exercises

Seated Arm Lifts

Areas Targeted: Shoulder, upper arm, back, abdomen muscles, and proprioception.

1. Sit upright in a chair with your feet hip-width apart.

2. Spread your knees slightly to allow your hands to touch the flat section of the seat in front of you.

3. Cup your right hand with your left hand and, with both hands together slowly raise your arms in front of you and then up over your head.

4. Slowly lower your arms.

5. Then raise them again. This time, keep them pointing forward but move slightly out to the side. Ending with your hands in the air above your head approximately in line with your right shoulder so that your back is curved slightly to the right.

6. Slowly lower your arms and then repeat, aiming to end with your arms above your head approximately in line

with your left shoulder and your back slightly curved to the left.

7. Repeat this set of three times for a total of eight.

If you are struggling when you first start, you can make this exercise easier by only raising your arms halfway. If necessary, you can aim to only reach the height of your shoulders. Try to avoid twisting your torso. The aim is to keep your shoulders facing forwards as you lift your arms.

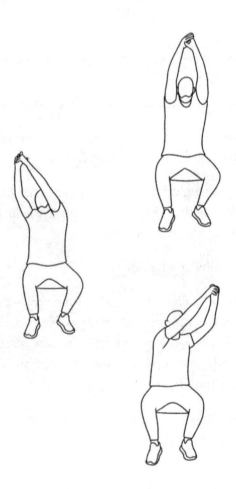

Cup Toe Tap

Areas Targeted: Hips, abdomen, thigh muscles, and proprioception.

1. Place a cup on the floor in front of you, in line with the middle of your chair.

2. Sit upright in your chair and tuck your heels in towards the front legs of the chair.

3. Lift your right leg and move it into the center tapping your toes on top of the cup.

4. Return your right leg back to the ground in front of the chair leg.

5. Lift your left leg and move into the center tapping your toes on top of the cup.

6. Return your right leg to the ground in front of the chair leg.

7. Alternate each leg until you have completed eight taps on each side.

Try to avoid moving your legs too far away from your cup or out to the side whenever you return your foot to the ground. Also, be sure that your cup is centered in front of you. You can make this exercise easier or more difficult by lowering or raising the height of the cup that you choose.

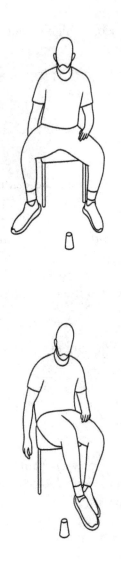
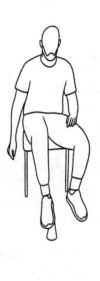

Seated Arm and Leg Lifts

Areas Targeted: Hips, thighs, abdomen, back, shoulder muscles, coordination, and proprioception.

1. Sit in your chair with your feet hip width apart.

2. Raise your right arm and right leg at the same time, keep your arm straight and your leg bent at the knee at 90 degrees.

3. Lower your right arm and right leg at the same time, then swap sides.

4. Raise your left arm and left leg at the same time, keep your arm straight and your leg bent at the knee at 90 degrees.

5. Lower your left arm and left leg.

6. Continue alternating each side of your body until you have completed eight lifts on each side.

If you find it too difficult to alternate from side to side, you can make this exercise a little easier by completing eight repetitions on one side first and then switching to do eight repetitions on the other. Aim to lift your arm right up above your head and bring your knee as close to your chest as you can manage. Avoid allowing your torso to bend to the side or allowing your body to tip over to the side that you are currently raising in the air.

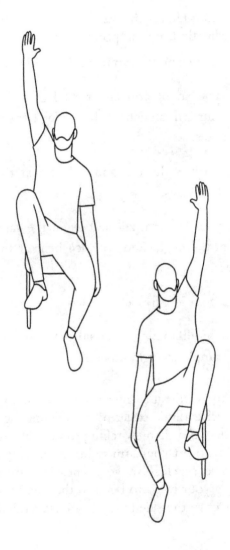

Torso Rotation Leg Openers

Areas Targeted: Hips, abdomen, back, thigh, buttocks muscles, and proprioception.

1. Sit upright in your chair with your feet hip apart.

2. Slide your left leg out to the side of the chair until your legs are at right angles to one another at the hip.

3. Then twist your torso to the right so that you are feeling a light stretch around your left hip area.

4. Twist your torso back to the center then return your left leg to its resting position in front of you.

5. Slide your right leg out to the side of the chair until your legs are at right angles to one another at the hip.

6. Then twist your torso to the left so that you are feeling a light stretch around the right hip area.

7. Twist your torso back to the center and then return your right leg to its resting position in front of you.

8. Continue alternating from side to side until you have completed eight twists in either direction.

Aim to twist your torso so that you can look over the back of the chair. It is fine if you cannot twist this far when you are first starting out. If you are finding this exercise difficult, you can support your upper torso by placing your arms on your extended knee and the back of the chair for support. However, avoid using your arms to pull your body into a twist. The movement should come from your hips and spine only. You may experience pain in your inner hip, especially if you stand or sit still for long periods of time. If this is the case, you can reduce the intensity by either reducing the degree of your torso rotation or by sliding your leg a shorter distance, thus reducing the angle between your legs.

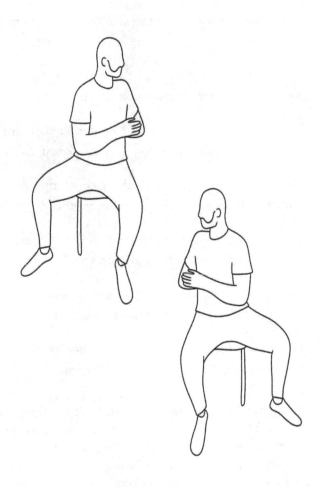

Forward Reach to the Ankle Tap

Areas Targeted: Hips, abdomen, back, shoulders, buttocks, thighs, and calf muscles; coordination; visual input; and proprioception—particularly the balance structures in the ear.

1. Sit upright in your chair with your feet hip width apart.

2. Slide your right foot forwards, straightening your leg and keeping the sole of your foot flat on the floor.

3. With your left arm, reach forward and over your center to touch the inside of your right ankle.

4. Return to an upright position then slide your right foot back towards the chair.

5. Slide your left foot forwards, straightening your leg and keeping the sole of your foot flat on the floor.

6. With your right arm, reach forward and over your center to touch the inside of your left ankle.

7. Return to an upright position then slide your left foot back towards the chair.

8. Continue alternating from side to side until you have completed eight ankle taps on each side.

You may experience some pain at the back of your knee, in your calves, or hamstrings if you are used to standing still a lot. To reduce this, you can reduce the distance that you slide your feet away from the chair and keep your knees slightly bent. And when you lean forward, be sure that most of the movement is happening at your hips and try to avoid curling your spine over your knee.

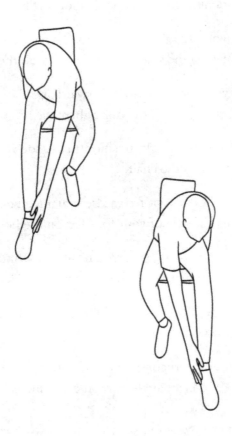

Chapter 5:

Standing Exercises

Side Leg Raise

Areas Targeted: Hips, abdomen, back, buttocks, outer thigh muscles, coordination, visual input, and proprioception.

1. Stand with your feet hip width apart.

2. Place your hands on your waist with a bend at your elbows.

3. Lift your right leg out to the side keeping your knee straight.

4. Then lower your right leg back to the floor.

5. Lift your left leg out to the side keeping your knee straight.

6. Then lower your left leg back to the floor.

7. Continue alternating sides until you have completed eight raises with each leg.

Your torso will naturally lean a little to the opposite side of the leg that you are raising. However, be sure not to allow yourself to bend sideways at the waist. Also, avoid allowing your torso to lean so far that you feel you will topple over. If you are finding this difficult, you can perform this exercise standing in front of a kitchen counter, which you can hold for support.

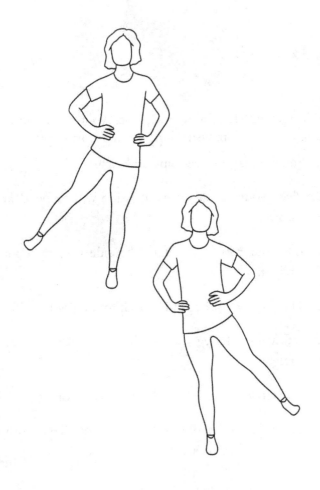

Forward Heel Taps

Areas Targeted: Hips, ankles, knees, back muscles, coordination, visual input, and proprioception.

1. Stand with your feet hip width apart and your arms at your sides.

2. Step forwards with your right foot allowing only the heel to make contact with the floor.

3. Return your right foot to your original hip width stance.

4. Then step forward with your left foot allowing only the heel to make contact with the floor.

5. Return your left foot to your original hip width stance.

6. Continue alternating feet until you have completed eight heel taps on each side.

Aim to keep your ankle bent so that your toes point slightly upwards when you tap your heel on the floor. However, the more that you bend your ankle upwards, the more difficult this exercise will become. If you are finding this difficult, you can moderate the exercise by taking smaller steps or, if need be, by touching your heel to the opposite toes only and then returning to your hip width stance. And you can also perform this exercise standing next to a wall facing sideways onto it so that when you step forward you do so parallel to the wall and can support yourself by placing your hand against the wall.

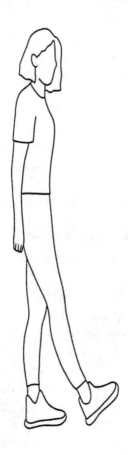

Side Toe Taps

Areas Targeted: Hips, knees, ankles, abdomen, back, buttock muscles, coordination, visual input, and proprioception.

1. Stand with your feet hip width apart and your hands at your sides.

2. Step out to the side using your right foot.

3. Allow your left knee to bend so that your right step can be larger, tap your right toes to the floor at your side.

4. Bring your right foot back into your hip width stance.

5. Then step out to the side using your left foot allowing your right knee to bend so the step can be larger.

6. Bring your left foot back into your hip width stance.

7. Continue alternating sides until you have completed eight toe taps on each side.

Remember that the larger you make your steps, the lower you will need to dip by bending your opposite knee and the more difficult this exercise will become. In the beginning, if you are finding this exercise too difficult, you can stand in front of a kitchen counter and hold onto it for support. While doing this exercise, remember to keep your back straight and do not allow yourself to bend over towards either side.

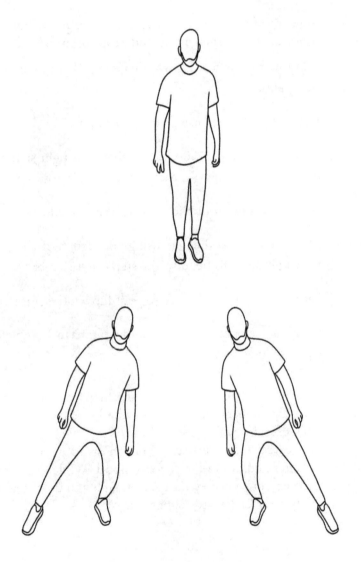

Heel Raise

Areas Targeted: Ankles, knees, buttocks, calf muscles, and proprioception.

1. Stand with your feet hip width apart behind the back of a chair.

2. Hold the back of your chair with both hands for support.

3. Raise both heels off the floor at the same time until you are on your tiptoes.

4. Then lower your heels back to the ground.

5. Repeat this process 10 times.

If you are finding this exercise difficult, you can reduce the height that you raise your heel from the ground. For safety reasons, I recommend a chair be used for this exercise. Aim to keep your ankles, knees, and hips in a straight line up from the floor. By this, I mean avoid allowing your joints to bow out to the sides or into the middle whilst you raise your heels.

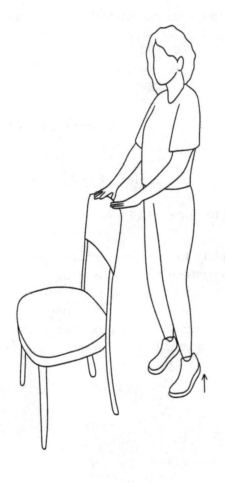

Toe Raise

Areas Targeted: Ankles, knees, buttocks, calf muscles, and proprioception.

1. Stand with your feet hip width apart behind the back of a chair.

2. Hold the back of the chair with both hands for support.

3. Raise the balls of your feet on both sides at the same time so that you are lifting your toes towards the ceiling.

4. Lower your toes back to the floor.

5. Repeat this process 10 times.

You may find that you bend slightly at the hip to allow yourself to continue holding the back of the chair. A small bend is fine, but avoid a tendency to squat downwards. If you are finding this exercise difficult, remember that the higher you lift the toes, the harder it will become. Therefore, you can reduce the intensity when you first begin by doing smaller sized toe raises.

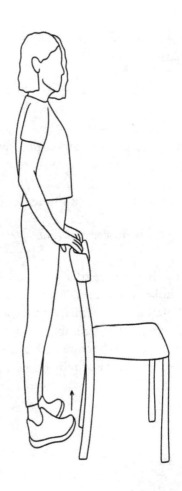

Lean Forward

Areas Targeted: Hips, abdomen, back, and shoulder muscles; coordination; visual input; and proprioception—particularly the balance structures in the ear.

1. Stand with your feet hip-width apart.

2. Touch the inside edges of your wrists together with your fingers pointing forwards and raise your arms out in front of you until they are level with your shoulders.

3. Lean your torso forward until your shoulders cross an imaginary line made by the front of your toes.

4. Stand back upright and pause.

5. Then lean forwards again and repeat the lean eight times.

The further forwards that you lean the more off center your weight will be balanced and the more difficult the exercise will become. Remember that your hips might bend slightly backwards while you do this. A small bend is fine, but avoid allowing your hips to take over the motion. You want to reach forward and not squat backwards. If you are finding this exercise too difficult, you can adapt it by completing the leans without your arms stretched in front of you.

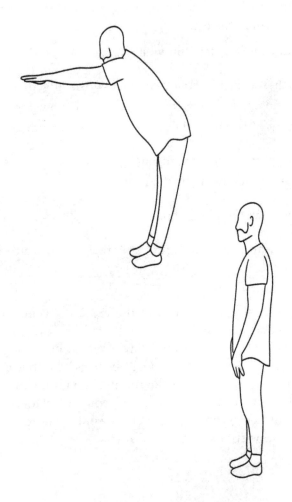

Side Lean

Areas Targeted: Hips, abdomen, back, shoulders, and muscles at the sides of the chest; coordination; visual input; and proprioception—particularly the balance structures in the ear.

1. With your feet hip width apart and your arms at your sides.

2. Raise your left arm out to your left side until it is parallel to the floor.

3. Then lean your torso towards your left.

4. Stand back upright then lower your arm.

5. Switch sides to raise your right arm until it is parallel with the floor.

6. Lean your torso towards the right.

7. Stand back upright then lower your arm.

8. Continue alternating sides until you have completed eight leans on each side.

Remember that when you lean to the side, you should be bending your spine, allowing your hips to bend out backwards. If you are finding this exercise too difficult, you can moderate the complexity by completing the side lean without your arms stretched out to the side.

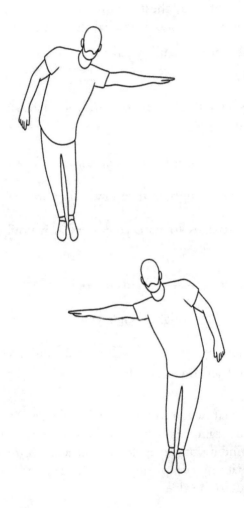

Tandem "Side to Side"

Areas Targeted: Ankles, hips, abdomen, back, neck muscles, visual input, and proprioception.

1. Stand with your feet one in front of the other, touching the heel of your front foot to the toes of your back foot. It doesn't matter which foot is in front you can choose whichever is most comfortable.

2. Keep your arms by your side and turn your head to face the left until you are looking over your left shoulder.

3. Turn your head back to the center and then turn your head to the right until you are looking over your right shoulder.

4. Turn your head back to the center so that you are facing forwards.

5. Keep alternating the side that you look at until you have turned each way eight times.

Try to avoid allowing your torso to twist. The aim of this exercise is to turn your head so that you are looking away from the direction that your body is pointing. If you are finding this exercise difficult, you can begin by standing sideways parallel to a wall and supporting yourself with one hand on the wall. If you experience vertigo, you might find this exercise particularly difficult. However, if you do not experience any dizziness, it is fine for you to still practice this movement.

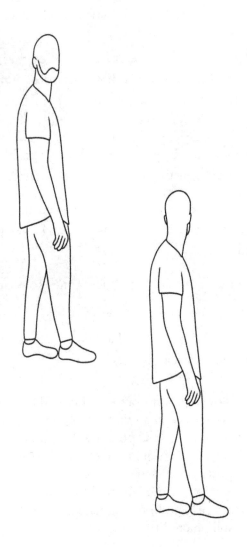

Rock the Boat

Areas Targeted: Ankles, knees, hips, abdomen, and back muscles; coordination; visual input and proprioception—particularly the balance structures in the ear.

1. Stand with your feet shoulder width apart.

2. Keeping your hands at your sides, lift your left foot off the ground keeping your knee straight and allowing your weight to rock over onto your right leg.

3. Rock back onto your left leg as you return your foot to the floor, then lift your right leg allowing your weight to transfer to your left.

4. Continue alternating sides until you have completed eight rocks in each direction.

The aim of this exercise is that you keep your back straight and do not bend to lean to the side. Rather, what you are looking for is a stiff looking movement that resembles that of a rocking chair, the exception being that this movement is side to side rather than backwards and forwards. When you lift your leg, raise it as far as you can from the ground without losing your balance. If you are finding this exercise difficult, you can adapt it by reducing the height to which you lift your legs.

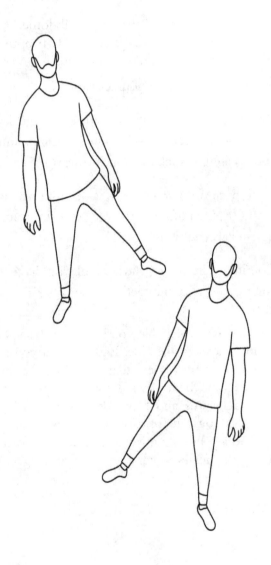

A Giant Backwards Step

Areas Targeted: Ankles, knees, hips, abdomen, back, thigh, and calf muscles; coordination; visual input; and proprioception—particularly the balance structures in the ear.

1. Stand with your feet hip width apart.

2. Place your hands on your waist with your elbows bent.

3. Step backwards on your left foot. Make the step as large as possible, bending the right knee to accommodate the large distance of the backward step.

4. Return your left foot to your resting hip-width position.

5. Step backwards onto your right foot, bending your left knee to allow you to make as large a step as possible.

6. Return your right foot to your resting hip-width position.

7. Continue alternating each side until you have completed eight giant steps with each leg.

Aim to keep the front leg pointing forwards and avoid allowing your knee to tip outwards to the side. Be sure to securely plant the ball of your back foot on the ground as you take your giant backward step. You don't want to touch the top of your foot to the floor, as this may over stretch your ankle. If you are finding this exercise difficult, you can reduce the intensity by taking smaller steps. However, this will also reduce the effectiveness, so I recommend only doing this for a few sessions and gradually increasing the size of your steps as you go along.

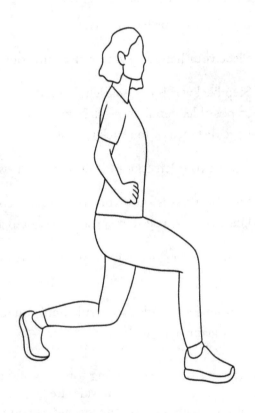

Chapter 6:

Walking Exercises

Tightrope Walk

Areas Targeted: Ankles, knees, hips, abdomen, and back muscles; visual input; coordination and proprioception.

1. Stand straight with your arms at your sides.

2. Move your left foot in front of your right foot, touching your left heel to your right toes, forms a straight line forward with both feet.

3. Next, move your right foot to step in front of your left. Touch your right heel to your left toes.

4. Continue stepping forward, one foot in front of the other until you have achieved 20 steps.

The aim is to walk in as straight a line as possible while keeping your balance. Imagine that you are walking on a tightrope or that you have a line painted on the floor that you must follow, like a sobriety test. You can look at your feet to help you get the placement correct, but over time, the aim would be to be able to walk 20 steps with your head held high, looking forward. If you find this exercise particularly difficult, you can perform it by walking alongside your kitchen counters so that you have a surface to hold onto if you are feeling unsteady.

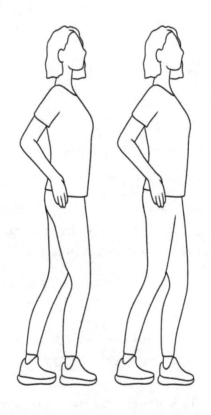

High Knee Marches

Areas Targeted: Ankles, knees, hips, thighs, buttocks, abdomen, and back muscles, visual input, and proprioception.

1. Stand straight with your arms at your sides.

2. Raise your left leg in the air, bending at least 90 degrees at both the hip and knee.

3. Place your left foot down in front of you.

4. Transfer your weight to your left leg and swap sides.

5. Raise your right leg in the air, bending at least 90 degrees at both the hip and knee.

6. Place your right foot down in front of you.

7. Walk forwards raising your knees as high as you can before setting your feet down onto the floor in front of you with each step.

8. Continue repeating this exaggerated step, alternating the leg that you step forward with until you have completed 20 steps.

The aim of this exercise is to practice balancing for a longer time on one leg while still moving forward. It will develop your ability to confidently make large strides when walking on slopes, upstairs, or anywhere else that there is uneven ground. Try to raise your knees as high as you can and keep looking ahead as you march. There is no need to swing your arms, but if you find it helpful in the beginning, you can do so. Just remember that you don't want the momentum of your arms to pull you along. As with the tightrope walk, if you are finding this difficult, it is okay to perform alongside the line of your kitchen counters for security.

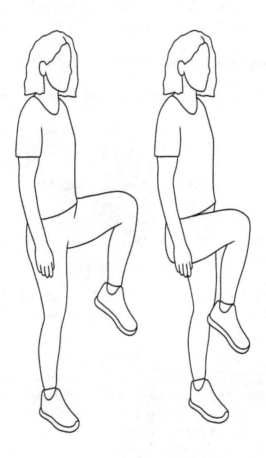

Crossovers

Areas Targeted: ankles, knees, hips, thighs, buttocks, abdomen, and back muscles; visual input; coordination; and proprioception.

1. Stand straight with your feet hip-width apart.

2. Cross your left leg in front of your right leg, stepping your foot out to your right side.

3. Then follow with your right leg to the right, undoing the crossing of your legs as you do so.

4. Step your left leg to the right again this time crossing your leg behind your right leg.

5. Undo the cross of your legs once more by stepping your right leg out to the right side.

6. Then reverse your direction of travel. Start by crossing your right leg in front of your left leg and out to your left side.

7. Uncross your legs by stepping your left leg out to the left.

8. Cross your legs again by passing the right leg behind your left leg to step to the left.

9. Uncross your legs by stepping your left leg out to the left side.

10. Repeat this pattern of crossing and uncrossing your legs until you have achieved the full motion four times in

irection, creating eight crossovers with one leg in
\d eight crossovers with one leg behind.

This exercise is very similar to a dance move that is sometimes known as the 'grapevine.' Its intention is for you to practice switching your weight from one leg to the other in more than one plane of movement, without necessarily traveling forward. This will help you get used to keeping stable when walking on uneven surfaces, as well as practice training your brain to recognize where your feet are in the space around you. If you are finding this exercise difficult, you can perform it in front of a wall so that you can reach out to support yourself if needed. Try to avoid looking down at your feet, as this can disorientate you since you're making an unusual pattern of steps.

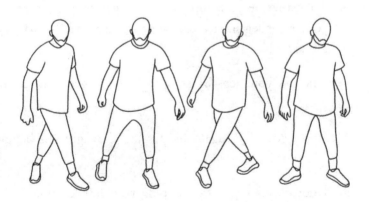

Sidesteps

Areas Targeted: Ankles, knees, hips, thighs, and buttock muscles; visual input; and proprioception.

1. Stand with your feet hip-width apart.

2. Move your left leg out to the side, creating a wide sidestep, notice that your body will become closer to the ground to account for the new wider stance.

3. Bring your right leg to meet your left leg so that you are standing upright with your feet hip-width apart again.

4. Repeat the step to the left re-making a wide stance and then closing the stance by bringing your right foot in to meet your left foot.

5. Now switch directions. Move your right leg out to the side making a wide stance and allowing your body to dip again.

6. Bring your left leg in to meet your right and stand upright again.

7. Repeat the step to the right, remembering to make a wide low stance allowing your body to dip.

8. Repeat two steps to the left and two steps to the right, alternating each direction until you have achieved 20 steps each way.

This exercise will raise and lower your center of gravity as you move, which will help you to practice the motions that you would need to move between sitting and standing, as well as train your ability to duck away from objects, or gently reach for things in a cupboard. If you find this exercise difficult, it can be performed alongside some kitchen counters so that you are able to reach out and support yourself if you feel that you are going to lose your balance. Try not to look at your feet as you move from side to side; instead, keep your gaze ahead of you. This helps to train the balance center of your brain to understand sideways movement when taken in the context of your forward vision.

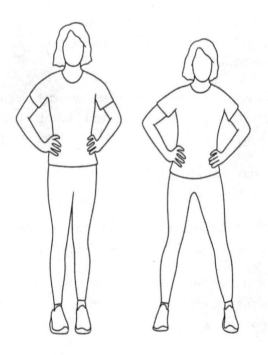

Heel Walks

Areas Targeted: Ankles, knees, hips, and calf muscles; visual input; and proprioception.

1. Stand straight with your feet hip-width apart and your arms at your sides.

2. Lift the balls of both feet off the ground, pointing your toes upwards.

3. Holding your toes off the ground, step forward with your left foot first. Use only your heels to make contact with the floor as you move.

4. Repeat the forward step walking onto your right heel with your toes still in the air.

5. Continue walking one foot in front of the other with only your heels making contact with the floor. Walk this way until you have achieved 20 steps—10 on each foot.

This exercise can be quite demanding, so if you are finding it difficult, you can walk alongside a wall, placing your hand against it for assistance. Keeping your toes pointing upward at all times is the aim. The movements in this exercise can be especially challenging for those who spend a lot of time sitting, and can feel uncomfortable at the back of their calves. At first, you may also feel wobbly. This is fine as long as you do not feel any dizziness. If you experience pain or sudden dizziness, stop immediately and rest.

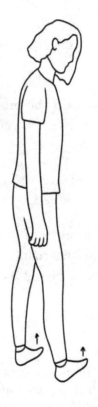

Toe Walks

Areas Targeted: Ankles, knees, hips, and calf muscles; visual input; and proprioception.

1. Stand straight with your feet hip-width apart and your arms at your sides.

2. Rise onto your toes so that the balls of your feet are the only parts of your feet touching the ground.

3. Walk forward, left foot first. Ensure that your heels do not touch the ground as you plant your feet on each step.

4. Repeat the forward step walking onto the toes of your right foot, with your heels still in the air.

5. Continue walking one foot in front of the other with only the balls of your feet making contact with the floor. Walk this way until you have achieved 20 steps— 10 on each foot.

If you regularly wear high heels, then this might be a familiar feeling for you. However, with this exercise, you do not have the support of the artificial heel and you will need to work on keeping your heels off the ground. This exercise strengthens the muscles at the back of your calf, which you use to propel yourself forward when walking normally. If you are finding this difficult, you can perform your toe walks alongside a wall so that you can reach your arm out to it for support. This exercise reduces the amount of contact that you have with the floor and challenges your balance centers to keep you steady with a limited area to transfer your weight through. This mimics walking on uneven terrain, stepping down steps, or as mentioned, wearing heels.

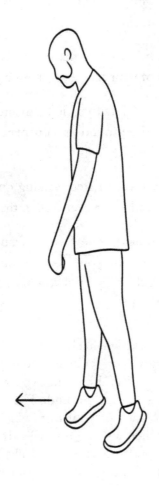

Figure Eight Walking

Areas Targeted: Ankles, knees, hips, abdomen, and back muscles; visual input; coordination; and proprioception—particularly the balance structures in the ear.

1. Place two paper cups on the ground roughly four feet apart.

2. Stand next to the cups so that they form a line traveling away from your side. Choose a location or object in front of you to keep your eyes focused on and continue looking at this spot throughout the exercise.

3. While keeping your eyes focused ahead of you, walk in front of the cup closest to you.

4. Step sideways around the first cup, and then backwards through the gap between the two cups.

5. Step sideways again to travel behind the second cup.

6. Loop around the outside of cup two and then in front of it, now traveling in the opposite direction to that in which you started.

7. Step backwards through the gap between the two cups, and then around the back of the first cup.

8. Continue walking in a figure of eight pattern in front of, between, and behind the two cups until you have completed five circuits around the cups in each direction.

By keeping focused on one spot with your eyes, you are practicing the ability for your brain to understand where your body is in relation to the space around you, as well as developing your ability to maintain your balance through steps in multiple directions. If you are finding this exercise difficult, there are a couple of ways that you can modify it:

- The first is that you can begin by looking in the direction that you are traveling while you walk around the cups rather than maintaining your chosen visual spot. This is a temporary measure and you should aim to be able to complete the figure of eight while looking in only one direction over time.

- If you have no problem maintaining your visual focus but still feel unsteady, you can replace the cups with two dining chairs. This will allow you to reach out and support yourself by holding the backs of the chairs while you are completing the steps. This will increase the size of your figure of eight, so you may also want to reduce the number of circuits that you complete when you begin this way.

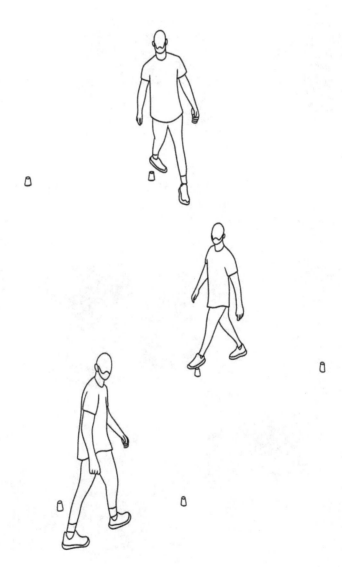

Chapter 7:

Core Exercises

You may have heard people talking about their core muscles before, as it is a very common part of most exercise routines. But something that is less often explained is why these muscles are important for injury prevention, pain reduction, and crucial for maintaining a healthy balance. Your core muscles consist of all the muscles within your pelvis and trunk, supporting your back and stabilizing your posture. These muscles are split into two groups:

1. The inner core, which consists of the muscles that support your spine, some span between your back bones, and others join your pelvis or ribs to your spine, will often be referred to as "core stability exercises."

2. The outer core, which consists of the muscles in your back and around your abdomen that are responsible for the movements generated in your torso, is the one that does the work of bending, twisting, or lifting things. Exercises targeted at this area are often referred to as "core strength exercises."

Having a healthy core system of muscles, both inner and outer, can reduce the onset of chronic back pain, provide your torso with healthy posture, and reduce the likelihood of trips and falls. The balance centers in the brain that rely on proprioception require both core strength and core stability to function correctly to properly understand and control the position of your body in relation to your limbs and anything that is around you.

A Russian Twist

Areas Targeted: Hips, thighs, buttocks, abdomen, back, core, and upper arm muscles; visual input; coordination; and proprioception—particularly the balance structures in the ear.

1. Sit on the floor with your knees bent and your heels touching the ground.

2. Clasp your hands together and lean backward slightly. You need to create enough space between your torso and knees so that you can easily pass your joined hands between them.

3. Twist your torso to the left, placing your hands in the space between your knees and abdomen, then keep twisting to reach your hands out to your left side and towards the ground.

4. Then twist your torso to the right, bringing your hands back to the center and then out to the right towards the ground.

5. Continue twisting, alternating left to right, for 20–40 seconds.

This exercise can be very challenging for anyone who has low core strength, so if you are finding it too difficult in the beginning, don't get discouraged. Adapt the exercise to suit your needs until you are confident enough to perform it fully.

To adapt, reduce the amount of lean that you start with. If it is particularly hard for you, you can start by sitting completely upright and twisting from side to side to touch the floor. You will need to lower your knees to be able to do this. Over time, slowly introduce an element of learning and increase the amount a little each time you come back to this exercise.

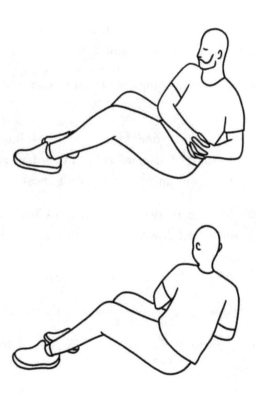

Hollow Crunch

Areas Targeted: Hips, thighs, buttocks, abdomen, back, core, shoulder, and upper arm muscles; visual input; coordination; and proprioception—particularly the balance structures in the ear.

1. Lay on the floor with your legs out straight and your arms by your sides.

2. Raise your arms over your head and bring them back down to the floor above you.

3. Next you need to complete two movements at the same time:

    o   Movement one: raise your legs into the air, bending 90 degrees at both your hips and knees, tuck your knees towards your chest.

    o   Movement two: lift your arms back over your head and down to your sides, as you bring your arms towards your sides curl your shoulders up off the floor to meet your chest to your knees.

4. Lower your legs and raise your arms above your head.

5. Keep repeating the whole movement for 20–40 seconds.

The aim is to complete the full movement in a slow, controlled manner, avoiding swinging your arms or grabbing onto the sides of your legs to pull yourself forward. Your shoulders and head should raise up off the ground, but you aren't trying to achieve a sit up, instead the goal is to bring your rib cage towards your hips. You can adapt this exercise to make it easier if you are a beginner to core exercises by sitting in a chair and curling your back forwards to bring your ribs down towards your hips.

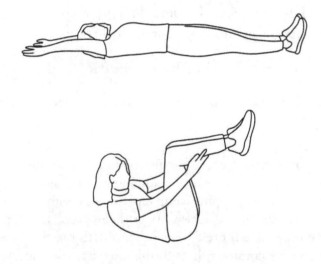

Single Leg Lifts

Areas Targeted: Hips, thighs, buttocks, abdomen, back, core muscles, and proprioception.

1. Lay on the floor with your legs straight and your arms by your sides.

2. Lift your left leg into the air, keeping your knee straight and bending your hip to 90 degrees.

3. Lower your left leg back to the floor.

4. Lift your right leg into the air, keeping your knee straight and bending your hip to 90 degrees.

5. Lower your right leg back to the floor.

6. Continue raising your legs, alternating one at a time for 20–40 seconds.

Tuck your tummy towards the floor while you do this exercise, you don't want to hold your breath, but create a tension in your abdomen. Avoid gripping your hips or legs with your hands while you do this exercise. If it helps you to stop this temptation, you can press your palms flat to the floor instead. Once you are comfortable with this exercise, you can increase the intensity by lifting your head and shoulders off the floor. This creates a mini crunch as you work.

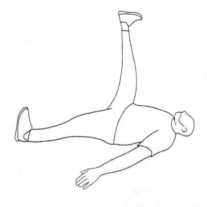

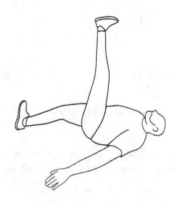

Mountain Climbers

Areas Targeted: Hips, thighs, buttocks, abdomen, back, core, shoulder, and upper arm muscles, coordination, and proprioception.

1. Start by leaning forward on your hands and knees, then straighten your legs out behind you so that the balls of your feet are making contact with the floor.

2. Keep your arms straight at the elbow and your palms flat on the floor at roughly shoulder-width apart.

3. Bend your left leg at the knee and hip, bringing it forward underneath you so that you mimic the starting position of an athletics race.

4. Straighten your left leg again and switch sides.

5. Bend your right leg at the knee and hip, bringing it forwards underneath you.

6. Straighten your right leg again and switch sides.

7. Continue alternating legs for 20–40 seconds.

Be sure to keep your upper back as straight as possible while doing this exercise. A small curl in your lower back is normal, however, as you tuck each knee up towards your chest. Another thing that it is important to avoid is allowing your elbows to twist inwards or outwards, as this can cause unnecessary strain on the joint. The higher you tuck your knees, the more effective this exercise will be.

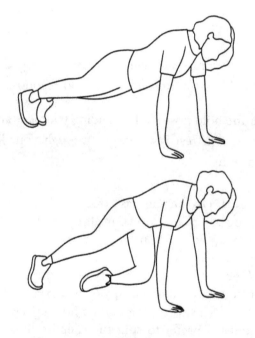

Plank

Areas Targeted: Hips, thighs, buttocks, abdomen, back, core, shoulders, and upper arm muscles, and proprioception.

1. Start by leaning forward on your hands and knees, bend your arms at the elbow and rest your forearms along the floor so that your weight is on your elbows.

2. Straighten your legs out behind you, resting your weight on the balls of your feet.

3. Tuck in your abdomen by gently tensing the muscles and holding this position for 20–40 seconds.

4. Exit the hold position by bending your legs at the knees and hips to rest your weight through your knees, and then sit up.

The plank is a challenging task for any beginner to core exercise, so you can adapt it to yourself by reducing the amount of time that you hold the position. Start with as low as 10 seconds and gradually increase your hold as you become more practiced. Once you are comfortable achieving 40-second holds, you can increase the intensity of this exercise by bending your knees to take a short rest and then holding again for up to three repetitions. I prefer to split the exercise into reps rather than increase the length of hold past 40 seconds, as a longer hold increases the temptation to bend at the hips, which reduces its effectiveness and activates the wrong muscles.

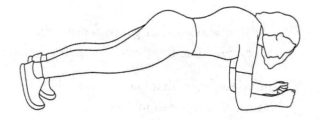

Side Plank

Areas Targeted: Hips, thighs, buttocks, abdomen, back, core, shoulder, and upper arm muscles, and proprioception.

1. Lay on your left side on the floor with your legs straight.

2. Lift your torso off the floor with one arm, leaning your weight through your elbow with your forearm lying flat across the floor pointing in front of you.

3. Lift your hips upwards to create a straight line with your body.

4. Tuck in your abdomen by gently tensing the abdominal muscles and holding this position for 20–40 seconds.

5. Exit this position by first lowering your hips back to the ground and then your shoulders.

6. Switch sides and repeat on your right side, holding for 20–40 seconds.

It is important to remember to tuck in your abdomen as activating these muscles will provide support to your lower back while you perform this exercise as well as increase the effectiveness of this position. Avoid the temptation to allow your hips to dip, creating a curve in the line of your body. Instead, aim to keep an imaginary line from your head, along your spine, and down your legs to the floor as straight as possible. As with the plank, I recommend adding extra repetitions with rests in between if you feel confident in increasing the intensity of your side planks.

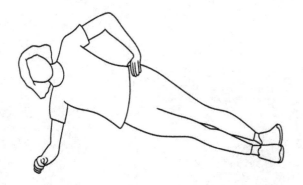

Chapter 8:

Vestibular Exercises

What Is Vestibular Exercise?

Vestibular exercises are a unique sub-set of exercises targeted specifically at training the balance centers in your brain and nervous system. The goal of these exercises is to challenge your brain to reinterpret its memory of how balance works for you. Over time, vestibular routines will reprogram the balance center of your brain to compensate for any injuries, abnormalities in the nervous system, or other contributors to poor balance that you may have. The overall outcome of these routines is that you will experience improved spells of dizziness, improved posture and stability within each posture, improved stability of your gaze while moving, and ultimately an improved quality of life due to gaining confidence in yourself that you can move about safely and without fear of falling.

Vestibular exercises will focus on training your gaze stability, hand-eye coordination, and correcting any compensations that you may be making due to an existing ailment in your balance centers; reducing the effects of aging on your ability to balance; and improving your ability to remain stable with multi-directional movements.

Each exercise will challenge the point at which you experience dizziness. For that reason, it is normal to feel some dizziness when you start. You will then work on that point of activating dizziness to push it back and become more confident. However, if you experience anything more than mild dizziness or discomfort, you should stop immediately and consult your health practitioner. Like any exercise aimed at strengthening muscles, vestibular exercises work best when consistently repeated and gradually increased in intensity. In the beginning, you may want to be sure that you practice these exercises with surfaces nearby that you can hold onto for support if you feel overwhelmed. If you have an existing balance disorder such as vertigo, you may also want to start these exercises with someone else present to help you.

ZigZag Walking

Areas Targeted: Hips, thighs, buttocks, abdomen, and back muscles; visual input; coordination, and proprioception.

1. Start in an area where you have plenty of space in front of and to the side of you.

2. Stand with your feet hip width apart and your hands at your sides.

3. Choose a location on the wall opposite you, or an item at the far end of the room and keep your gaze fixed on that location or item.

4. Walk forward in a diagonal line to your left.

5. Once you reach the opposite side of your exercise space, change directions so that you are walking in a diagonal line to your right. Remember to keep your gaze fixed on your chosen location while you are

walking, this will result in your head turning to the side as you walk.

6. Continue switching directions until you have completed five diagonal walks in each direction.

If you have limited space, you can still do this exercise by completing one or two diagonal walks and then going back to your starting position to do more. The key to this exercise being successful is to maintain your gaze position throughout. You will be training your body to understand how movement feels when it is occurring in a direction at odds with your vision and to strengthen its ability to maintain posture and stability when doing so. Don't be afraid to take a rest in between each zigzag set if you need to. You want to avoid pushing yourself until you are dizzy or faint.

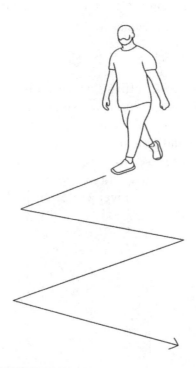

Eyes Side to Side

Areas Targeted: Facial muscles around the eyes, visual input, and proprioception.

1. Stand straight with your feet hip-width apart for stability.

2. Hold your arms still and point your head directly forward.

3. Look to your left as far as you can move your eyes only.

4. Then switch directions and look to the right as far as you can without moving your head.

5. Keep alternating the direction that you move your eyes until you have achieved 15 sets of looking in each direction.

If you find this exercise difficult or have a history of falls, you may wish to begin by training your eye movements while sitting and gradually move on to being able to complete this while standing. You should aim to keep your head facing forward throughout this exercise to train your balance center to interpret your surroundings and understand that movement of the gaze doesn't equate to movement of the body.

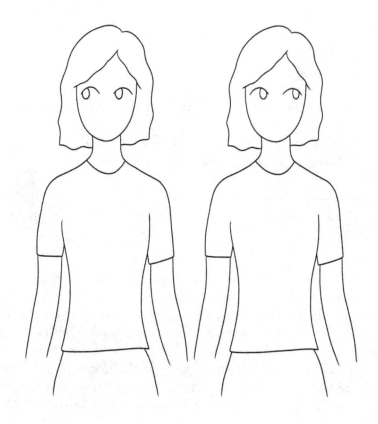

Eyes Up and Down

Areas Targeted: Facial muscles around the eyes, visual input, and proprioception.

1. Stand straight with your feet hip-width apart for stability.

2. Hold your arms still and point your head directly forward.

3. Look upwards as far as you can move your eyes only.

4. Then switch directions and look downwards as far as you can without moving your head.

5. Keep alternating the direction that you move your eyes until you have achieved 15 sets of looking up and down.

As with the eyes side to side exercise, if you are a beginner or have previously experienced falls, you may wish to start this exercise in a seated position first. Once you are more confident, you can build up to doing this in a standing position. Looking up can be particularly difficult if you suffer from vertigo or other balance disorders linked to the balance center. If this is the case for you, you may want to conduct these exercises in front of a kitchen counter so that you can hold onto it for support.

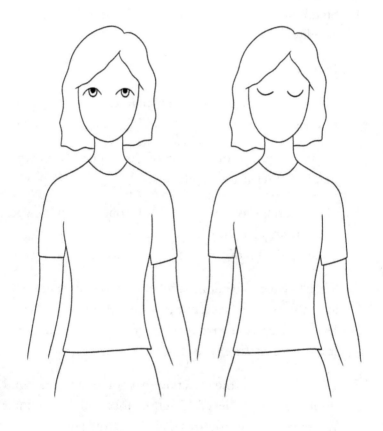

In and Out

Areas Targeted: Facial muscles around the eye, shoulder, and upper arm muscles, visual input, coordination, and proprioception.

1. Stand straight with your feet hip-width apart for stability.

2. Point your head directly forward.

3. Lift one arm and use your pointer finger to point towards the ceiling.

4. Focus your gaze on the tip of your finger while your hand is at full arm's length.

5. Slowly bring your hand toward your face until your pointer finger is touching your nose. Keep your gaze fixed on the tip of your finger as it moves towards you.

6. Then switch directions and slowly move your hand away from your face until it is once again at full arm's length. Keep your gaze fixed on the tip of your finger as it moves away from you.

7. Keep alternating the direction that you move your hand until you have achieved 15 sets of focus on your pointer finger as it moves towards and away from you.

Remember to move your arm in a slow, steady line to and from your face. If you do this too quickly, it can increase the tendency to only focus on the beginning and end positions of your finger, forgetting all the distance in between. If you have any existing visual impairments that you have been prescribed glasses to correct, you will want to be sure that you have these on during this exercise to avoid causing a headache.

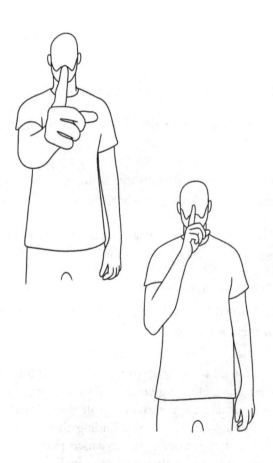

Head Up and Down

Areas Targeted: Neck and back muscles, visual input, and proprioception—particularly the balance structures in the ear.

1. Stand with your feet hip-width apart and your arms still at your sides.

2. The starting position for your head should be facing forward.

3. Tilt your head back to look up at the ceiling.

4. Then, bring your head back to its natural resting position.

5. Tilt your head downward, bringing your chin to your chest and looking down at the floor.

6. Then, bring your head back to its natural resting position.

7. Continue alternating between looking up to the ceiling and down to the floor until you have achieved 15 sets of this movement.

Be sure to look all the way up to the ceiling and then all the way down to the floor, allowing your head to follow the direction of your gaze, rather than moving your head first and then adjusting your vision. If you are finding this exercise difficult, you can adapt it by halving the distance that you move your head as you look up or down when you first begin. You can then slowly increase the distance that you look as you become more confident. If you have a history of falls, you may wish to perform this exercise while sitting in a chair until you are more confident, particularly while looking upwards.

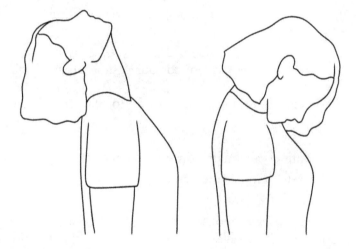

Head Side to Side

Areas Targeted: Neck and muscles, visual input, and proprioception—particularly the balance structures in the ear.

1. Stand with your feet hip-width apart and your arms still at your sides.

2. The starting position for your head should be facing forward.

3. Turn your head to look to your left as far as possible.

4. Then, bring your head back to its natural resting position.

5. Turn your head to look to your right as far as possible.

6. Then, bring your head back to its natural resting position.

7. Continue alternating directions until you have achieved 15 sets of looking left and right.

Aim to keep your motions smooth and steady as you change directions. Be sure to allow your head to follow the direction of your gaze, rather than moving your head first and then adjusting your vision. When you look from left to right, look as far in each direction as you can without twisting your torso. If you are finding this difficult or have a history of falls, you may wish to practice this exercise in a chair before you perform it while standing.

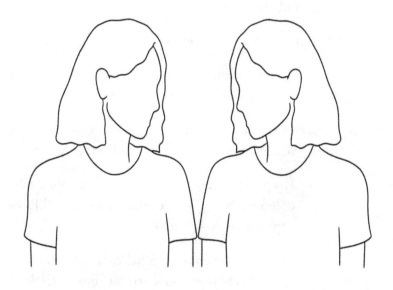

Sitting to Standing With Rotation

Areas Targeted: Legs and core muscles, visual input, coordination, and proprioception—particularly the balance structures in the ear.

1. Sit in a chair with your feet hip width apart.

2. Lean forward and plant your weight through your feet, then stand up.

3. Walk in a circle on the spot to your left:

   o Start by turning your left foot out to your side and transferring your weight to it.

   o Move your right foot next to your left, following through to turn your body.

   o Keep stepping this way until you have completed a full circle. This should be approximately 4–5 steps.

   o Once you have turned a full circle and you once again have your back to the chair, sit back down.

4. Repeat steps 1–4 until you have achieved five full sit-to-stand and rotations.

This exercise combines several skills that you may need to practice separately if you find it difficult to get into and out of chairs. If you are finding it particularly difficult, try placing your hands on your legs above your knees and pushing down through them as you stand. Alternatively, you could also swap your chair for one with arms built in and push down through those instead of placing your hands on your legs. Remember, though, if you switch your chair, that it still needs to have a solid base and back. Avoid using a recliner. It is normal when you begin to feel slightly dizzy while rotating your body on the spot. However, if this becomes disorienting or you feel lightheaded stop immediately. You should use extra caution in this exercise if you have vertigo or similar pre-existing balance disorders.

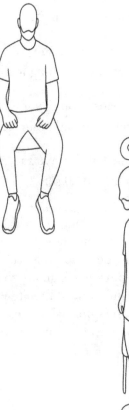
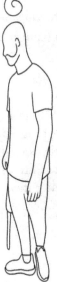

Ball Toss Head Height

Areas Targeted: Shoulder and arm muscles, visual input, coordination, reaction times, and proprioception.

For this exercise, you will need a small ball, like a ping-pong ball or a juggling ball.

1. Stand with your feet hip-width apart.

2. Lift both arms so that your elbows are bent and your hands are at the level of your face.

3. Hold the ball in your left hand then throw it from left to right in front of you, catching it with your right hand.

4. Throw the ball back from your right hand across in front of you, catching it with your left hand.

5. Keep throwing the ball from left to right and back again until you have achieved 20 sets.

Aim to keep your head facing forwards throughout this exercise. Try not to follow the direction that the ball travels. This exercise will help to develop your hand eye coordination, along with developing your brain's ability to locate the position of your hands precisely and rapidly. Don't worry if you find this exercise difficult at first. It is normal for this to require practice, and you will need patience to build up to 20 successful catches of the ball.

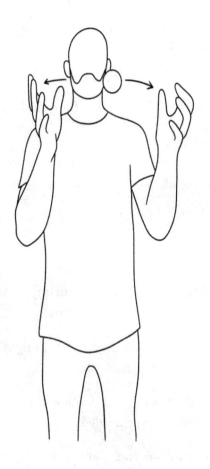

Ball Toss Between the Legs

Areas Targeted: Hips, thighs, buttocks, abdomen, back, core, and arm muscles; visual input; coordination; reaction times; and proprioception.

For this exercise, you will need a small ball, like a ping-pong ball or a juggling ball.

1. Stand with your feet hip-width apart.

2. Step forward on your left foot, and bend your knees slightly.

3. Lean forward so that your hands are below the level of your left thigh.

4. Hold the ball in your left hand then throw it from left to right between your legs, catching it with your right hand.

5. Throw the ball back from your right hand, under your leg, catching it with your left hand.

6. Keep throwing the ball from left to right and back again until you have achieved 10 sets.

7. Return to standing with your feet hip-width apart and take a short break if needed.

8. Step forward on your right foot, and bend your knees slightly.

9. Lean forward so that your hands are below the level of your left thigh.

10. Then repeat the process of throwing the ball from left to right underneath the front leg until you have achieved another 10 sets.

This exercise tests your balance from both a physical aspect, in your muscles' ability to hold the stance required, and a balance center perspective to train your coordination. If you are finding this exercise difficult, you can drop the knee of the back leg to the floor so that your shin is resting along the ground and your front leg is bent at 90 degrees at both the knee and hip. You can also practice the hand motions without the ball and then reintroduce the ball toss once you are confident that you can safely hold the stance required.

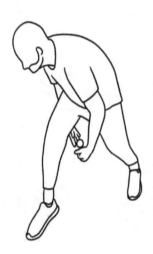

Chapter 9:

Advanced Balance Exercises

The exercises contained in this Chapter are very challenging. They combine multiple aspects of balance training and may need to be practiced in smaller sections before you put them all together as you become more confident. Remember to practice each exercise with caution. Training may feel uncomfortable, but it should never be painful. If you feel any pain, lightheadedness, or disorientation, then you should stop and consult with your primary physician or other health professional. Consider keeping a chair nearby or working out next to a kitchen counter that you can hold onto if you feel unstable at any point. You may also want to have someone with you to lend a hand if you become particularly dizzy.

Around the World

Areas Targeted: Ankles, knees, hips, thighs, buttocks, abdomen, back, and core muscles; visual input; coordination; and proprioception—particularly the balance structures in the ear.

1. Stand with your feet hip-width apart.

2. Bend your left leg at the knee to dip your body towards the ground as you reach your right foot forward and touch your right foot to the floor.

3. Straighten your legs and bring your right foot back in to join your left.

4. Bend your left leg again, this time reaching your right leg out to your right side and touch your foot to the floor.

5. Straighten your legs and bring your right foot back in to join your left.

6. Bend your left leg once more, reaching your right leg out behind you and touching your foot to the floor.

7. Straighten your legs and bring your right foot back in to join your left.

8. Keep your left leg straight and cross your right leg over in front of it, to tap your right foot to the ground at your left side.

9. Uncross your legs and bring your right foot back in to join your left.

10. Repeat this pattern until you have reached all four directions three times.

11. Once the three sets are completed, switch the leg that you are using to reach out with to your left leg.

12. Bend your right leg at the knee to dip your body towards the ground as you reach your left foot forward and touch your left foot to the floor.

13. Straighten your legs and bring your left foot back in to join your right.

14. Bend your right leg again, this time reaching your left leg out to your left side and bringing your foot to the floor.

15. Straighten your legs and bring your left foot back in to join your right.

16. Bend your right leg once more, reaching your left leg out behind you and touching your foot to the floor.

17. Straighten your legs and bring your left foot back in to join your right.

18. Keep your right leg straight and cross your left leg over in front of it, to tap your left foot to the ground at your right side.

19. Uncross your legs and bring your left foot back in to join your left.

20. Repeat this pattern until you have reached all four directions three times.

If you are finding it difficult to complete this exercise, you can reduce the distance from the body that you reach with the foot that you are moving in each direction. This will reduce the pressure on your weight bearing leg as you bend the knee. Similarly, if you have been practicing for a few weeks and are safely completing the full cycle with confidence, you can reach further away to dial up the difficulty of this exercise.

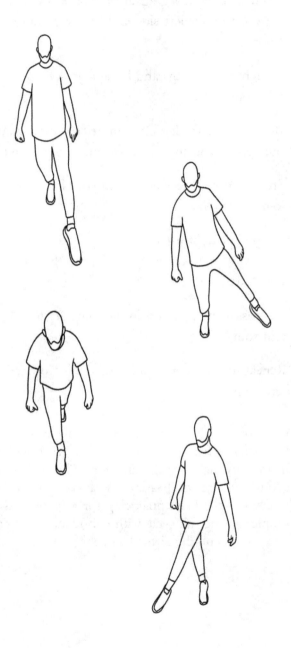

Tree Pose

Areas Targeted: Feet, ankles, knees, hips, thighs, buttocks, abdomen, back, and core muscles; visual input; coordination; and proprioception.

1. Stand with your feet hip-width apart and your arms at your sides.

2. Lift your left foot, bending your leg at the knee.

3. Place the sole of your left foot against the inside of your right leg with your toes pointing downward.

4. Hold this position for 20–60 seconds.

5. Place your left foot back on the ground.

6. Then, lift your right foot, bending your leg at the knee.

7. Place the sole of your right foot against the inside of your left leg with your toes pointing downward.

8. Hold this position for 20–60 seconds.

The goal when doing this exercise is to place the sole of your lifted foot above the knee of the opposite leg and keep your arms at your sides. If you are finding it difficult to get into the correct position, you can adapt the exercise by lowering your foot. The lower your foot, the easier the exercise will become. However, be sure never to place your foot directly against the opposite knee, to avoid placing unnecessary pressure on that joint. You can also raise your arms out to your sides so that they are level with your shoulders to help you maintain your balance until you are confident enough to keep them at your sides. In the beginning, aiming for a 20-second hold may seem like a challenge, and that is fine. You can increase the length of your pose each time you practice until you gradually reach 60 seconds.

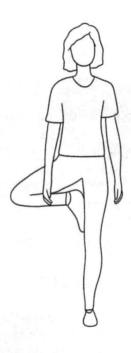

Front Scale

Areas Targeted: Ankles, knees, hips, thighs, buttocks, abdomen, back, core, shoulder, and upper arm muscles, visual input, coordination, and proprioception.

1. Stand with your feet hip-width apart and your arms at your sides.

2. Lift your left leg, bending only at the hip and hold it straight out in front of you.

3. Lift your arms out to your sides to help you maintain your balance.

4. Hold this position for 20–60 seconds.

5. Lower your left leg to the floor and switch sides.

6. Lift your right leg, bending only at the hip and hold it straight out in front of you.

7. Lift your arms out to your sides to help you maintain your balance.

8. Hold this position for 20–60 seconds.

Start by aiming to hold your pose for 20 seconds at a time. Then, gradually increase the length of time that you hold your position as you become more practiced, until you can confidently reach a 60-second hold. Once you are safely achieving 60-second holds on both legs, you can increase the intensity of the exercise by lowering your arms and aiming to achieve the hold with both arms resting at your sides. Conversely, if you are finding this exercise difficult, you can keep a chair at your side and reach out to hold it until your balance is strong enough for you to no longer need the support.

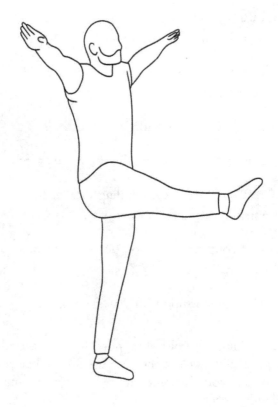

Back Scale

Areas Targeted: Ankles, knees, hips, thighs, buttocks, abdomen, back, and core muscles; visual input; coordination; and proprioception—particularly the balance structures in the ear.

1. Stand with your feet hip-width apart.

2. Lift your left leg out behind you and lean forward until you create a horizontal line along your back and down the length of your leg that is parallel to the floor.

3. Spread your arms out to the sides to help you maintain your balance.

4. Hold this pose for 20–60 seconds.

5. Lower your left leg back to the floor and stand upright, then switch sides.

6. Lift your right leg out behind you and lean forward until you create a horizontal line along your back and down the length of your leg that is parallel to the floor.

7. Spread your arms out to the sides to help you maintain your balance.

8. Hold this pose for 20–60 seconds.

As with the front lean, begin by setting yourself a target of 20 seconds for your hold time. Once you are comfortable with achieving this time on both sides, you can begin increasing your hold until you reach 60 seconds on each side. After you have achieved a full 60-second hold and are confident that you can safely begin to adapt to this exercise, you can make it more difficult by pulling your arms in toward your sides or holding them in front of your chest with your elbows bent. If you are finding this exercise difficult, you can keep a chair nearby so that you can hold it back while you practice, until you are safely able to hold the pose without needing the extra support.

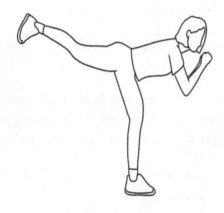

Chapter 10:

Different Tools for Balance

As with any form of exercise, you can assist your balance training by making use of specialist equipment. This doesn't mean that the equipment is difficult to source or that it must be prescribed by a health professional, but that it is designed specifically for the purpose of improving your ability to balance and creating a healthier balance center. There are many forms of equipment available on the market today, and it can be intimidating to search for something that suits your needs. In this Chapter, I break down four kinds of specialty equipment that I believe are the most effective in enhancing balance training routines.

Balance Board

Balance boards can be used to replicate a variety of situations where your balance will be tested. You use balance boards by placing them soft side down and standing on top, then adapting your movements each time the board moves to stay upright. By putting your body into these positions, you can train your ability to react appropriately to this kind of stimulus and improve your balance for many everyday activities. Balance boards usually consist of a soft base such as a rubber or plastic dome and a hard top surface that extends away from the base that you can stand on while you exercise. The boards are usually plastic or wood for strength so that they can easily hold your weight and are often used in rehabilitation classes following injuries.

While they started as a rehabilitation tool in therapy settings, there are many types of balance boards available on the market today for use at home:

1. **Traditional balance board**: Usually a wooden top surface with a soft cylindrical bottom that allows movement in a linear direction.

2. **Wobble board**: Can be plastic or wood but usually include a tough grip surface on top and a half ball shape underneath that gives free movement in 360 degrees around the center.

3. **Electronic balance boards**: These are plastic and usually consist of two flat surfaces separated by bars and push buttons that provide movement and resistance. They will provide feedback on your performance through a visual display, these can be expensive, but there are also some available that are designed to function with gaming consoles.

4. **Lateral slide boards**: These boards consist of two flat surfaces separated by bars. Unlike the electronic boards, these don't provide resistance and only have end bumpers to prevent the top board slipping off entirely. These are very challenging and are not recommended for beginners.

5. **Standing desk balance board**: These can provide linear or 360-degree movement but are generally a bit stiffer than other boards so that they are less mobile and able to be used for longer periods of time.

Using a balance board is an advanced way of pushing your balance training, so it is important that you start any exercise with this tool near to a surface you can hold for stability or with another person for support, until you become more adept at using the balance board. The movement of the balance board can be unpredictable, especially when you first start using it while your natural reaction to maintain your center of balance is likely compromised. The board will cause you to continually make corrections in your posture to remain upright, so it can be labor intensive. For this reason, you should begin with short sessions, aiming to remain balanced for 20–60 seconds. Once you achieve this safely, you can increase the amount of time that you spend using the balance board to suit your own goals. Some people even use them for long periods of time in front of a standing desk while they work.

After you become confident in standing on a balance board safely, you can challenge yourself by completing exercises while using the board. You can add in things like a squat or torso lean in any direction. You can also introduce the *Ball Toss Head Height* exercise featured in Chapter 8. There are many ideas easily found online for adapting your balance board routine. Try experimenting to find a challenge that you enjoy and that suits your own personal balance goals.

Bosu Ball

Bosu Balls were designed in 1999 by David Weck and the name stands for *both sides utilized* (Mead, 2022). It is a semi-sphere that resembles half of an exercise ball with a flat surface that does not significantly extend past the diameter of that ball half. When used with the flat side up, the bosu ball creates an unstable surface that can be utilized in the same way as a balance board, but when used with the flat side down, the ball becomes much more versatile. The flat surface against the ground creates a stable surface that isn't going to move while you exercise with it, but more uniquely, the upper curved surface, which is full of air like an exercise ball, provides a cushioned surface that you can use to train your balance while simultaneously lessening the load on your joints as you move through your exercises.

The curved surface of the bosu ball can be used to provide support for back and abdominal stretches that allow you to safely stretch further than you may be able to while sitting or standing. To take advantage of this, for example, you can train your core strength by laying on your side, placing your hips on top—but near to the edge—of the curved surface, creating an anchor for yourself against the floor by placing your legs roughly shoulder-width apart on the ground in front of each other. You can then lower your upper body over the curve of the bosu ball so that your shoulders move towards the floor, lifting your shoulders back up to create a curve in your spine in the opposite direction towards the ceiling. Complete 15–20 of these stretch combinations on each side. The ball can be used in this way for abdomen stretches; moving your shoulders towards the floor while laying on your back, combined with a mini crunch to lift your shoulders back up, or as a support for your feet while doing calf stretches—there are multiple videos available online giving inspiration for using the bosu ball as a stretching aid.

In addition to the advantages that the bosu ball brings in terms of active stretching, it can also be used flat side down to enhance your balance training. Standing on top of the curved surface barefoot can improve the way your brain processes feedback from the feet to make corrections in posture necessary to keep you stable. Another advantage to working on the bosu ball barefoot is that it will give you an opportunity to strengthen muscles in the foot that you wouldn't ordinarily use while wearing shoes but that play an important role in a healthy ability to balance. After some practice, once you are confident that you can stand on the curved surface safely, you can introduce some of the standing exercises in Chapter 5 while on the bosu ball. Exercises like toe taps, heel taps, and forward leans can be particularly effective when paired with this tool, as the bosu ball encourages activation of your whole core while progressing through them.

Balance Pad

Balance pads are square sponge or gel pads–usually around three inches thick–that create an unstable surface which can be stood on while exercising to encourage activation of muscles needed for stability. Unlike balance boards, they don't produce large movements that require a lot of adaptation in your posture to master. Because of this, they are great for beginners or anyone with a history of falls, ankle rolls, or pre-existing balance disorders. Balance pads are particularly useful for strengthening the muscles around your ankles and knees, though they also force you to practice your ability to process feedback from your feet to make body wide corrections to remain upright.

As a beginner's tool, a great way to get started is to stand with both feet on the pad and close one eye to see how this affects how stable your body feels. Do practice closing each eye and comparing them to see if you notice a difference between the left and right. Do you feel like you need to employ more corrections to your posture on one side than the other? It isn't unusual to feel a disparity between the two, especially if you have injured one leg or ankle in the past. For people who experience a lot of balance difficulties, this alone can be a challenging exercise, but once it is mastered, the balance pad can be used in many standing exercises to work the balance center and muscles simultaneously.

Some of my favorite exercise adaptations for the balance pad include:

- **Toe or heel raises; Chapter 5**: Stand central on the balance pad and perform the toe and heel raise to challenge your ankles and core.

- **High Knee Marches on the Spot; Chapter 6**: March on top of the balance pad to strengthen your legs and hips.

- **Sidesteps; Chapter 6**: Start on the bare floor next to the balance pad and sidestep onto it, then sidestep again off the other side. Practice both directions. This will encourage your balance center to process changing ground types as you move.

- **Russian twists; Chapter 7**: Sit on the balance pad to perform your twists. This will increase the work that your core must do to remain in the required pose and will increase the intensity of this exercise.

- **Plank or side plank; Chapter 7**: Rest your arms on the balance pad while doing these exercises to challenge your core in maintaining a straight spine.

- **Tree Pose, Chapter 9**: This exercise adaptation shouldn't be attempted by beginners. Be sure that you are confident in performing the tree pose on the bare ground before attempting to use the balance pad here. stand on top of the balance pad to practice this pose, try to keep the foot that you are standing on as close as possible to the center of the pad. This will challenge your balance center and whole body to maintain a stable position.

Stability Ball

The stability ball is an air-filled ball that comes in a variety of sizes and is also known as the "exercise ball," "swiss ball," or "physio ball." Like other equipment, it was initially used as a rehabilitation tool but has since been adopted by several gyms and is an inexpensive home exercise addition. Stability balls are the most readily available and accessible tool in this Chapter. They aren't recommended for standing but can replace a chair in any seated exercise to increase the effectiveness of that workout. Stability balls are hailed for their ability to improve posture and have even been taken into offices in place of regular chairs to facilitate the wellness of workers.

There is more than just good posture to be gained from the stability ball. However, like the other tools listed here, it forces your body to process feedback about its position and constantly adjust to remain stable, becoming an effective balance training aid. The key area of the body trained by the stability ball is the core. Muscles in the lower back are activated immediately to keep you in place when you sit on it. Additional benefits include reduced load on the joints in the same way that the bosu board cushions the body, improved reaction time, reduced back pain, and improved confidence in mobility.

Conclusion

Physical well-being necessitates listening to what you already know, and then taking it seriously enough to act accordingly. When you wake up and feel the impulse to arch your back, stretch and exhale with a loud sigh, for God's sake, do it. –Darrell Calkins

They say that the best time to start anything new was yesterday, but the second-best time is today. Now that you have access to a bank of well-rounded balanced targeted exercises, you can build your muscle coordination, improve your proprioception, strengthen your core, and feel confident in getting back out there to enjoy life without fear of falling.

Remember to set a regular time that suits you and commit to your routine. Consistent balance practice is key to really making the most of your exercises. You don't need to slog through the whole book every day; instead, complete your warm-up and choose ten exercises that will total around 15 minutes per day. Make sure you switch up your chosen exercises each time you workout to keep things enjoyable, and make sure you train your whole body. Preparing a plan of exercise rotations in advance can help to make sure that you don't miss out on any important tasks. This is why I created my weekly planner and made it available to you for free! I want to give you all the tools you need to succeed.

To receive your complimentary copy now, please visit *www.robertbalazs.com.*

This is also what drove me to create a book that is fully illustrated and to provide videos of each exercise being performed from start to finish. Everyone has a different way of learning and taking in information, so I wanted to make these exercises as accessible as possible no matter which style of learning suits you best.

To get your video companion playlist, please visit *www.tinyurl.com/Rob-Balazs*.

The exercise adaptations in this book are intended to make the exercises feasible for all ability levels, whether you have existing balance disorders or are recovering from an injury, or you consider yourself generally healthy but have noticed that your coordination isn't what it used to be. Remember, there are always ways to make the exercises easier on you when you are feeling out of your depth. You don't need to feel like balance training is too complicated or difficult for you. On the flip side, once you have been practicing for some time, you may feel like you want a bit more of a challenge, then it's time to embrace the advanced exercises and examine tools for balance training so that you can push yourself while working out.

We all know that you will be more disappointed by the things you didn't do than by the ones you did. Go for it! Enjoy every second of this journey and come back with a ton of amazing memories. –Unknown

You can look forward to better reaction times, coordination, and improved stability. So, what are you waiting for? There is no time like the present. Start your weekly planner and get on your way to a healthier balance today.

No matter where you start in ability level, I can't wait to see where your balance training journey takes you and would love to hear your feedback via reviews.

To leave a review, scan the QR code at the beginning of the book with your mobile phone and click on the book. Once you have clicked on the book, you will be able to find the button to leave a review. If you don't have a smartphone able to scan the

QR code, you can also access the reviews by searching for the book title again on Amazon.

References

Balance Problems: Basic Facts. (2022). AGS Health in Aging Foundation. https://www.healthinaging.org/a-z-topic/balance-problems/basic-facts

Back To Motion Physical Therapy. (n.d.). Importance of Balance Training for Seniors - Back To Motion. *Denver Physical Therapy. Back to Motion Physical Therapy.* https://backtomotion.net/importance-of-balance-training-for-seniors/

Bhupathiraju, S. (2022, April 7). 9 Best Vestibular Exercises. *Styles At Life.* https://stylesatlife.com/articles/vestibular-exercises/

Brennan, D. (2021, March 18). What Causes Balance Issues in Older Adults. *WebMD.* http://https_www.webmd.com/?url=https%3A%2F%2Fwww.webmd.com%2Fhealthy-aging%2Fwhat-causes-balance-issues-in-older-adults

Carroll, J. (2005, December 6). Regular Exercise: Who's Getting It? *Gallup News.* https://news.gallup.com/poll/20314/Regular-Exercise-Whos-Getting-It.aspx

Centers for Disease Control and Prevention. (2021, August 6). Facts About Falls. *Centers for Disease Control and Prevention.* https://www.cdc.gov/falls/facts.html

Dillon, C. F., Gu, Q., Hoffman, H. J., & Ko, C.-W. (2010, April). Vision, Hearing, Balance, and Sensory Impairment in Americans Aged 70 Years and Over: United States, 1999–2006. *NCHS Data Brief,* 31, 1-8.

Edwards, D. (2019, August 19). The Top 8 Benefits of Balance Training. *Primal Play.* https://www.primalplay.com/blog/8-benefits-of-balance-exercises

Elderly Fall Prevention. (2022). Choosing the Right Walking Aids. *Elderly Fall Prevention.* https://elderlyfallprevention.com/assistive-devices/walking-aids/

Elflein, J. (2021, February 16). • Prevalence of moderate or severe vision impairment by age and gender worldwide 2020. *Statista.* https://www.statista.com/statistics/1238083/prevalence-moderate-severe-vision-impairment-by-age-gender/

Fitness Drum. (2021, April 26). Balance Pad Exercises That Will Work Wonders For Your Stability and Body Control. *Fitness Drum.* https://fitnessdrum.com/balance-pad-exercises/

Fox, R. (2022, April 30). Why Balance Is So Important For Seniors (and How To Improve Yours). *Silver Fox Fitness.* https://gentlestrengthexercises.com/why-balance-is-so-important-for-seniors/

Freedom Care. (2020, June 24). Why Senior Citizens Should Perform Balance Exercises. *FreedomCare.*

https://www.freedomcareny.com/posts/why-should-senior-citizens-perform-balance-exercises

Gaspari Nutrition. (2019, July 10). What Are The Pros & Cons of BOSU Balls? *Gaspari Nutrition.* https://gasparinutrition.com/blogs/fitness-facts/what-are-the-pros-cons-of-bosu-balls

Han, B. I., Song, H. S., & Kim, J. S. (2011, December 29). Vestibular Rehabilitation Therapy: Review of Indications, Mechanisms, and Key Exercises. *Journal of Clinical Neurology, 7*(4), 184-196. 10.3988/jcn.2011.7.4.184

Huffman, M. (2015, May 14). Use of walking aids jumps 50% in 10 years. *ConsumerAffairs.com.* https://www.consumeraffairs.com/news/use-of-walking-aids-jumps-50-in-10-years-051415.html

Kinetix Physical Therapy. (2022). The Connection Between Core Strength and Better Balance. *Kinetix Physical Therapy.* https://kinetixpt.com/the-connection-between-core-strength-and-better-balance/

Konrad, H. R., Giradi, M., & Helfert, R. (1999, September). Balance and Aging. *The Laryngoscope, 109*(9), 1454-60. 10.1097/00005537-199909000-00019

Larsen, E. (n.d.). 4 Proven Benefits of Stability Ball Exercises: Science And Facts | FITNESS. *HomeTrainingHero.* https://www.hometraininghero.com/benefits-stability-ball-exercises-science-behind-effectiveness/

Leaf Group Ltd. (2022). Why You Should Train With a Balance Board and How to Get Started. *Livestrong.com.*

https://www.livestrong.com/article/34421-balance-board-benefits/

Mayo Clinic. (2020, August 29). Core exercises: Why you should strengthen your core muscles. *Mayo Clinic*. https://www.mayoclinic.org/healthy-lifestyle/fitness/in-depth/core-exercises/art-20044751

McKeon, P. O., & Hartel, J. (2008, May-June). Systematic review of postural control and lateral ankle instability, part II: is balance training clinically effective? *Journal of Athletic Training, 43*(3), 305-15. 10.4085/1062-6050-43.3.305

McKeon, P. O., Ingersoll, C. D., Kerrigan, D. C., Saliba, E., Bennett, B. C., & Hartel, J. (2008, October). Balance training improves function and postural control in those with chronic ankle instability. *Medicine and Science in Sports and Exercise, 40*(10), 1810-9. 10.1249/MSS.0b013e31817e0f92

Mead, T. (2022). What Is A Bosu Ball And How To Use It. *Alternative   Daily*. https://www.thealternativedaily.com/how-to-use-a-bosu-ball/

National Institute on Aging. (2022, June 16). Prevent Falls and Fractures | National Institute on Aging. *National Institute   on   Aging*. https://www.nia.nih.gov/health/prevent-falls-and-fractures

North Central Surgical Center. (2016, March 10). The benefits of exercising with a stability ball. *North Central Surgical*

Center. https://www.northcentralsurgical.com/blog/the-benefits-of-exercising-with-a-stability-ball-54.html

Rettner, R. (2016, July 8). Everything You Need to Know About Balance Exercise. *Live Science.* https://www.livescience.com/55321-balance-exercise.html

Smith, E. (2015, January 5). The Benefits of a Bosu Ball. *American Home Fitness.* https://americanhomefitness.com/blogs/news/the-benefits-of-a-bosu-ball

Techno Gym. (n.d.). Balance Pad: Exercises for Your Workout. *Technogym.* https://www.technogym.com/us/newsroom/balance-pad-exercises-workout/

University of Mississippi. (n.d.). Vestibular (Balance) Exercises. *University of Mississippi Medical Center.* https://www.umc.edu/Healthcare/ENT/Patient-Handouts/Adult/Otology/Vestibular_Exercises.html

U.S. Department of Health & Human Services. (2022, June 3). How much physical activity do older adults need? | *Physical Activity.* CDC. https://www.cdc.gov/physicalactivity/basics/older_adults/index.htm

CPSIA information can be obtained
at www.ICGtesting.com
Printed in the USA
LVHW040118110323
741363LV00006B/970